Digitised Health, Medicine and Risk

A prevailing excitement can be discerned in the medical and public health literature and popular media concerning the apparent 'disruptive' or 'revolutionary' potential of digital health technologies. Most of the wider social implications are often ignored or glossed over in such accounts. Critical approaches from within the social sciences that take a more measured perspective are important—including those that focus on risk. The contributors to this volume examine various dimensions of risk in the context of digital health. They identify that digital health devices and software offer the ability to configure new forms of risk, in concert with novel responsibilities. The contributions emphasise the sheer volume of detail about very personal and private elements of people's lives, emotions and bodies that contemporary digital technologies can collect. They show that apps and other internet tools and forums provide opportunities for health and medical risks to be identified, publicised or managed, but also for unvalidated new therapies to be championed. Most of the authors identify the neoliberal 'soft' politics of digital health, in which lay people are encouraged ('nudged') to engage in practices of identifying and managing health risk in their own interests, and the victim-blaming that may be part of these discourses. This book was originally published as a special issue of *Health, Risk and Society*.

Deborah Lupton is a Centenary Research Professor in the News & Media Research Centre, Faculty of Arts & Design, University of Canberra, Australia. Her research spans sociology and media and cultural studies. She is the author/co-author of 15 books and three edited volumes.

Digitised Health, Medicine and Risk

Edited by
Deborah Lupton

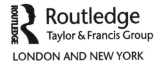

Routledge
Taylor & Francis Group

LONDON AND NEW YORK

First published 2017 by Routledge

2 Park Square, Milton Park, Abingdon, Oxfordshire OX14 4RN
711 Third Avenue, New York, NY 10017

Routledge is an imprint of the Taylor & Francis Group, an informa business

First issued in paperback 2018

British Library Cataloguing in Publication Data
A catalogue record for this book is available from the British Library

ISBN 13: 978-1-138-21362-3 (hbk)
ISBN 13: 978-0-367-02894-7 (pbk)

Typeset in TimesNewRomanPS
by diacriTech, Chennai

Publisher's Note
The publisher accepts responsibility for any inconsistencies that may have arisen
during the conversion of this book from journal articles to book chapters, namely
the possible inclusion of journal terminology.

Disclaimer
Every effort has been made to contact copyright holders for their permission to
reprint material in this book. The publishers would be grateful to hear from any
copyright holder who is not here acknowledged and will undertake to rectify any
errors or omissions in future editions of this book.

Contents

CONTENTS

Citation Information

The chapters in this book were originally published in *Health, Risk and Society*, volume 17, issues 7–8 (October–November 2015). When citing this material, please use the original page numbering for each article, as follows:

Introduction
Digitised health, medicine and risk
Deborah Lupton
Health, Risk and Society, volume 17, issues 7–8 (October–November 2015) pp. 473–476

Chapter 1
The gamification of risk: how health apps foster self-confidence and why this is not enough
Antonio Maturo and Francesca Setiffi
Health, Risk and Society, volume 17, issues 7–8 (October–November 2015) pp. 477–494

Chapter 2
Threats and thrills: pregnancy apps, risk and consumption
Gareth M. Thomas and Deborah Lupton
Health, Risk and Society, volume 17, issues 7–8 (October–November 2015) pp. 495–509

Chapter 3
Asthma on the move: how mobile apps remediate risk for disease management
Alison Kenner
Health, Risk and Society, volume 17, issues 7–8 (October–November 2015) pp. 510–529

Chapter 4
Digital 'solutions' to unhealthy lifestyle 'problems': the construction of social and personal risks in the development of eCoaches
Samantha Adams and Maartje Niezen
Health, Risk and Society, volume 17, issues 7–8 (October–November 2015) pp. 530–546

Chapter 5
Digitalised health, risk and motherhood: politics of infant feeding in post-colonial Hong Kong
Sau Wa Mak
Health, Risk and Society, volume 17, issues 7–8 (October–November 2015) pp. 547–564

CITATION INFORMATION

Chapter 6

Chapter 7

Chapter 8

For any permission-related enquiries please visit:
http://www.tandfonline.com/page/help/permissions

Notes on Contributors

Samantha Adams is an Associate Professor in the Tilburg Institute of Law, Technology and Society, Tilburg University, Tilburg, The Netherlands.

S. Fiona Barker is a researcher in the Faculty of Medicine, Nursing & Health Sciences, Monash University, Australia.

Mette Kragh Furbo is a Senior Research Associate in the Department of Sociology, Lancaster University, Lancaster, UK.

Barbara Hunter is a Senior Research Fellow in the Faculty of Medicine, Nursing & Health Sciences, Monash University, Australia.

Alison Kenner is an Assistant Professor in the Department of Politics, Drexel University, Philadelphia, USA.

Dan I. Lubman is a Professor at the Eastern Health Clinical School, Faculty of Medicine, Nursing & Health Sciences, Monash University, Australia.

Deborah Lupton is a Centenary Research Professor in the News & Media Research Centre, Faculty of Arts & Design, University of Canberra, Australia.

Casimir MacGregor is a Research Fellow in the School of Social Sciences, Monash University, Victoria, Australia.

Adrian Mackenzie is a Professor in the Department of Sociology, Lancaster University, Lancaster, UK.

Sau Wa Mak is a Lecturer in the Department of Anthropology, The Chinese University of Hong Kong, Shatin, New Territories, Hong Kong.

Antonio Maturo is an Associate Professor in the Department of Sociology and Business Law, University of Bologna, Bologna, Italy, and the Sociology Department, Brown University, Providence, USA.

Maggie Mort is a Professor in the Department of Sociology, Lancaster University, Lancaster, UK.

Megan Munsie is an Associate Professor at Stem Cells Australia, Department of Anatomy and Neuroscience, University of Melbourne, Australia.

Maartje Niezen is an Assistant Professor in the Tilburg Institute of Law, Technology and Society, Tilburg University, Tilburg, The Netherlands.

NOTES ON CONTRIBUTORS

Alan Petersen is a Professor in the School of Social Sciences, Monash University, Victoria, Australia.

Celia Mary Roberts is a Senior Lecturer in the Department of Sociology, Lancaster University, Lancaster, UK.

Michael Savic is a researcher in the Faculty of Medicine, Nursing & Health Sciences, Monash University, Australia.

Francesca Setiffi is a researcher in the Department of Political Science, Law and International Studies, University of Padova, Padova, Italy.

Gareth M. Thomas is a Lecturer in Sociology at the School of Social Sciences, Cardiff University, Cardiff, UK.

Joann Wilkinson is a PhD candidate and Associate Lecturer in the Department of Sociology, Lancaster University, Lancaster, UK.

INTRODUCTION

Digitised health, medicine and risk

The domains of medicine and public health have witnessed a rapid expansion of digital technologies over the past decade. While telehealth and telemedicine and patient online discussion forums were introduced in the 1990s in the wake of personal computing and the development of the Internet, the advent of mobile ubiquitous devices, apps and social media networking sites has resulted in a proliferation of opportunities for people to seek out information about health and medicine, share their experiences and collect their own biometric data. Healthcare professionals and public health workers, for their part, can employ digital technologies for professional and patient education and as part of their applied practice (see overviews of the range of technologies available in Lupton, 2014b, 2015).

A prevailing excitement can be discerned in the medical and public health literature and popular media concerning the apparent 'disruptive' or 'revolutionary' potential of digital health technologies. For example, glowing descriptions of the value of 'prescribing' apps to patients, encouraging people to share their experiences on social media and specialised platforms such as PatientsLikeMe, using big data to develop greater insights into patterns of health and illness, sending people with chronic health conditions home with wireless digital devices for self-care, employing 3D-printing technologies to manufacture prostheses or human tissue, educating medical students using iPads and virtual reality software and using wearable devices and apps for health promotion are common in these literatures.

There is no doubt that these technologies offer many possibilities for improving or enhancing healthcare, preventive health and public health. However, most of the wider social implications are often ignored or glossed over in such accounts. Critical approaches from within the social sciences that take a more measured perspective are important – including those that focus on risk.

Researchers in the social science of risk have various perspectives to offer on digital risk society in general (Lupton, 2016) and digital health technologies more specifically. Among other topics, they can seek to identify the socio-economic disadvantage or inequalities that digital health technologies may exacerbate or generate; show how the digital media represent risk discourses (on websites, Wikipedia, online news reports and social media platforms, for example); highlight the ways in which such technologies as apps and other software identify, algorithmically calculate, perform and manage some phenomena as 'health risks'; and uncover the unintended consequences for both laypeople and health professionals of using digital health technologies in healthcare and public health.

This special issue was designed to encourage social researchers' attention on these issues. Eight articles are included from authors addressing a range of issues concerning digitised health, medicine and risk. Several authors concentrate on apps: Samantha Adams and Maartje Niezen write about eCoaches (online health promotion software and related mobile apps) as they are used as part of a Dutch public–private programme, Antonio Maturo and Francesca Setiffi discuss the gamification of risk in weight-loss apps, Gareth Thomas and myself address the representation of risk and commodity consumption in pregnancy apps and Alison Kenner analyses the content, development and use of asthma apps. In their article, Maggie Mort and colleagues describe their study investigating how members of a north English community responded to two forms of biosensors for health monitoring: home ovulation and direct-to-consumer genetic testing technologies.

The exchange of information on online forums, blogs, social media sites and websites are examined in two articles. Alan Peterson, Casimir MacGregor and Megan Munsie provide an analysis of how social media were employed by patients to advocate for access to stem cell therapies. Sau Wa Mak's article discusses how Hong Kong mothers used social media and websites to learn about, gain support for and defend their infant feeding practices. Both articles emphasise the great importance that such digital media can have in facilitating lay discussion of health risks and in configuring new forms of biosociality and biological citizenship. Finally, the study reported by Michael Savic and colleagues addresses an Australian online screening intervention for alcohol and other drug-related harms. They identify the ways in which this software enacts certain behaviours and people as 'risky'.

All authors here published adopt an approach that recognises apps and other software, as well as hardware such as wireless patient self-care devices and wearable health and fitness trackers as sociocultural artefacts (Lupton, 2014a). Most of the analyses identify the neoliberal 'soft' politics of digital health, in which laypeople are encouraged ('nudged') to engage in practices of self-management and self-care in their own interests, and the victim-blaming that may be part of these discourses.

As a collection, the articles also highlight the sheer volume of detail about very personal and private elements of people's lives, emotions and bodies that contemporary digital technologies can collect: including their alcohol and drug use, physical activity, genomic information, infant feeding and care practices, medical treatments, eating habits, fertility, reproduction and sexual activity. A dominant feature of these technologies is their 'pushiness'; their tendency to use push notifications and warnings tailored to users' personal details for maximum effect. With their data-collecting capacity, these devices and software offer the ability to configure new forms of risk, in concert with novel responsibilities.

One important aspect of risk in relation to digital health that has not been addressed by the articles in the special collection is that relating to how people's often very private and intimate data about their bodies and behaviours have become exploited by others. The sharing economy of new digital media encourages people to upload their personal information to public forums as part of constructing identity and engaging in social relationships (Banning, 2015). However, people lose control of these details once they are uploaded to proprietary apps and platforms, and they become open to use by many different actors and agencies. In the new knowledge economy, personal digital data have become highly valuable for commercial, research, managerial, governmental and fraudulent purposes. A new digital divide has begun to emerge, in which the Internet empires and other large corporations have ownership of people's personal data while the public has limited access to their own data (Andrejevic, 2014; Fuchs, 2014).

Commercial organisations use the data that they gather from people's online transactions and app use to target them with advertising, or sell the data to third parties (Andrejevic, 2014). The use of personal data by third parties is beginning to have significant implications for people's life opportunities. Data mining companies use personal details that they can scrape from digital datasets (including their health and medical details) to construct profiles about people that may be used to limit their access to insurance, credit, employment and social security benefits (Crawford & Schultz, 2014;

Rosenblat, Wikelius, Boyd, Gangadharan, & Yu, 2014). Another risk relates to how certain social groups are excluded from big datasets because they do not engage in the activities that tend to routinely collect personal data via interactions with digital technologies. These groups tend to be already disadvantaged and marginalised, and this may be exacerbated when government and commercial entities rely on digital data to provide services and shape policy (Lerman, 2013).

A further personal data risk relates to data privacy and security. Data breaches and leakages are common in healthcare organisations and developers' archives of personal data, including those generated by health and medical apps (McCarthy, 2013; Wicks & Chiauzzi, 2015). Digital datasets on personal health and medical details have become a target of cyber criminals, who are able to use this information to profit from identify theft and fraud (Ablon, Libicki, & Golay, 2015).

Before his death, the late Ulrich Beck, a key figure in risk sociology, had begun to comment on what he termed 'global digital freedom risk' in the wake of the Snowden revelations of national security agencies' surveillance of their citizens' interactions online and private telephone records (Beck, 2013). This risk, for Beck, involved not only the threat to privacy, and free speech and communication posed by these security agencies but also the Internet empires. He emphasised the fundamental right of citizens to protect the privacy of their personal data. These issues require continuing attention from critical social researchers.

While this special issue has gone a small way towards contributing to the literature on the social dimensions of digitised health, medicine and risk, many other avenues remain open for exploration. Despite the very common use of social media sites such as Facebook, YouTube, Tumblr and Twitter for the communication of health and medical risk, surprisingly little sociological investigation has been undertaken of these sites. Even though there are now well over 100,000 health and medical apps available for both laypeople and healthcare professionals (Jahns, 2014), few social researchers have directed their attention at analysing the content of these apps and identifying how people are using them (or, why they choose *not* to use them). We know little, as yet, about the rationales and decision-making that underpin health policymakers and digital health developers, or the ways in which citizens are using apps and sensors as part of 'citizen science' public health initiatives. Given the rapidly changing environment of digital health, including new technologies such as apps, 3D-printing, sensor-embedded 'smart' objects and physical spaces and the emerging Internet of Things (in which smart objects communicate directly with each other), there is a panoply of potential topics to explore.

References

Ablon, L., Libicki, M., & Golay, A. (2015). *Markets for cybercrime tools and stolen data*. Santa Monica, CA: RAND Corporation.

Andrejevic, M. (2014). The big data divide. *International Journal of Communication*, 8, 1673–1689.

Banning, M. E. (2015). Shared entanglements – web 2.0, info-liberalism & digital sharing. Information, Communication & Society, *19*(4), 1–15.

Beck, U. (2013). The digital freedom risk: To fragile an acknowledgement. *OpenDemocracy*. Retrieved from https://www.opendemocracy.net/can-europe-make-it/ulrich-beck/digital-freedom-risk-too-fragile-acknowledgment

Crawford, K., & Schultz, J. (2014). Big data and due process: Toward a framework to redress predictive privacy harms. *Boston College Law Review*, *55*(1), 93–128.

Fuchs, C. (2014). *Social media: A critical introduction*. London: Sage.

Jahns, R.-G. (2014). The 8 drivers and barriers that will shape the mHealth app market in the next 5 years. *research2guidance*. Retrieved from http://mhealtheconomics.com/the-8-drivers-and-barriers-that-will-shape-the-mhealth-app-market-in-the-next-5-years/

Lerman, J. (2013). Big data and its exclusions. *Standford Law Review Online*. Retrieved from http://www.stanfordlawreview.org/online/privacy-and-big-data/big-data-and-its-exclusions

Lupton, D. (2014a). Apps as artefacts: Towards a critical perspective on mobile health and medical apps. *Societies, 4*(4), 606–622. doi:10.3390/soc4040606

Lupton, D. (2014b). Critical perspectives on digital health technologies. *Sociology Compass, 8*(12), 1344–1359. doi:10.1111/soc4.12226

Lupton, D. (2015). Health promotion in the digital era: A critical commentary. *Health Promotion International, 30*(1), 174–183. doi:10.1093/heapro/dau091

Lupton, D. (2016). Digital risk society. In A. Burgess, A. Alemanno, & J. Zinn (Eds.), *The Routledge handbook of risk studies* (pp. 301–309). London: Routledge.

McCarthy, M. (2013). Experts warn on data security in health and fitness apps. *British Medical Journal, 347*(f5600). Retrieved from http://www.bmj.com/content/347/bmj.f5600

Rosenblat, A., Wikelius, K., Boyd, D., Gangadharan, S. P., & Yu, C. (2014). Data & civil rights: Health primer. *Data & Society Research Institute*. Retrieved from http://www.datacivilrights.org/pubs/2014-1030/Health.pdf

Wicks, P., & Chiauzzi, E. (2015). 'Trust but verify': five approaches to ensure safe medical apps. *BMC Medicine, 13*(1), 205. doi:10.1186/s12916-015-0451-z

Deborah Lupton
News & Media Research Centre, Faculty of Arts & Design,
University of Canberra, Canberra, Australia

The gamification of risk: how health apps foster self-confidence and why this is not enough

Antonio Maturo[a,b] and Francesca Setiffi[c]

[a]Department of Sociology and Business Law, University of Bologna, Bologna, Italy; [b]Sociology Department, Brown University, Providence, RI, USA; [c]Department of Political Science, Law and International Studies, University of Padova, Padova, Italy

Weight loss apps enable users to quantify many aspects of food consumption, beginning with calories intake. Users of weight loss apps can also participate in online forums that act as digital self-help groups. These apps also include several features related to game playing or gamification such as avatars, points and virtual awards. Gamification has the aim of strengthening motivation to carry out a (boring) task. We downloaded the 20 most popular free weight loss apps in Google Play. We analysed app descriptions provided by developers, comments about the selected apps in online forums and user reviews. We focused on four of these apps, since they had some special functions. We found that users' risk management was based on a mixed method that combined quantification and gamification, that is, rationality and emotions. Quantification, which includes self-tracking, data analysis and graphic layout, provides the 'rational' basis for dietary regimes, while gamification provides the emotional support needed to maintain motivation and continue with the diet. Our analysis provides support for the emotion–risk assemblage theory and the in-between strategy. Our analysis reinforces the importance of emotions in risk management. However, these dieting apps are based on a reductionist approach to obesity and weight loss, as obesity is framed as an individual problem, while weight loss is seen as dependent on individual motivation. Such framing tends to conceal the social determinant of health and the social and political causes of obesity.

Introduction

In this article, we explore the ways in which weight loss apps frame the risks of obesity and structure individuals' responses to being overweight. Using data from an analysis of the 20 most popular dieting apps in the Google Play store, we demonstrate that these apps frame obesity as an individual risk, downplaying the social determinants of health and how other aspects of biopolitics are marginalised in the digital health realm.

Health apps and risk

Health apps

The authors of the European Commission's 'Green Paper on mobile health' (European Commission, 2014) outlined their high expectations for the potential of health apps. They noted that m-health could increase rates of early disease detection, reduce the cost of unnecessary consultations, increase prevention, contribute to a more sustainable and efficient health-care system and possibly foster patient empowerment. They also observed that almost 100,000 health- and well-being-related apps already exist. They called for further research in the areas of motivation and user engagement.

The development of m-health has been stimulated by the development of smartphones such as Apple's iPhone over the past decade. These new phones have become a powerful tool for the self-tracking and measurement of a wide range of activities such as sport performance, physiological states, behaviours and feelings. They enable individuals to collect and carry out a statistical analysis of huge amounts of information about themselves and then share these data with a wide audience on social networks. This capacity to capture, analyse and share data on individual's own behaviour, physiological states and performance has created a new culture of self-monitoring and personal analytics (Ruckenstein, 2014) that is supported and encouraged by online communication through digital platforms and social networks.

These new technological opportunities have stimulated a consumer-centred model of health, based on self-determination and 'the central role of patients in making decisions about the course of the care' (Guseva, 2013, p. 1). As the sources of medical information shift from those controlled by doctors such as medical records and specialist journals to interactive websites and online communities, it is easier for individuals and patients to find information, get support and share their illness experiences with others with the same conditions (Light & Maturo, 2015). These changes, among other factors, have also contributed to increasing expectations of health self-management and patient health literacy – though the information individuals may access online may not be subject to the same level of scrutiny and quality control as, for example, the findings reported in peer-reviewed journals.

This emphasis on individual or self-led healthcare is reflected in health apps that seek to tap into and enhance user motivation. These apps provide facilities for, inter alia, the keeping of digital diaries and the sharing of results with one's online community of 'friends'. Some features of apps are based on cognitive psychology approaches, such as the Transtheoretical Model of Health Behavior Change (Prochaska & Velicer, 1997), for behavioural changes such as quitting smoking or stopping drinking.

While the new technologies embedded in apps make it possible to monitor virtually any aspect of life, also work productivity for example, bodily functions remain the privileged target for self-tracking (Lupton, 2013b). This privileging is reflected in the large number of apps for losing weight – obesity is indeed increasingly labelled as one the most dangerous health problems in the world. For example, two-thirds of Americans are obese or over-weight (Flegal, Graubard, Williamson, & Gail, 2005). In the last 40 years, the number of obese people has tripled, while the number of overweight people has not changed (Sullivan, 2010). Given the wide array of weight loss-focused apps and the prevalence of overweight and obesity, we have focused our research on apps aimed at weight loss.

In our analysis, we focus on quantification; a social phenomenon that is growing in social life and as such should be studied through sociological concepts. The force of numbers in and of themselves has been of little interest to sociology in the past, possibly because quantification was so ubiquitous as to be taken for granted by laypeople and researchers alike. Health apps allow people to quantify any kind of experience and to create personal analytics. Alongside quantification, we will also discuss gamification, a technique intended to foster productivity and achieve goals by transforming work into a game. Most health apps (and many marketing strategies) are based on this strategy. Moreover, through their managerial language and graphics, these apps depict the user as a self-entrepreneur who works on herself as if she were an enterprise with the mission of increasing physical, cognitive and emotional 'productivity'.

The algorithmic body and the quantified self

Espeland and Stevens call for a sociology of quantification, claiming that quantification should be taken into consideration as a sociological phenomenon:

> Quantification is a constitutive feature of modern science and social organization, yet sociologists have generally been reluctant to investigate it as a sociological phenomenon in its own right. (Espeland & Stevens, 2008, p. 402)

Although there has been sociological interest in quantification, most of the discussion has focused mainly on the epistemological aspects of quantitative methods of social research (Bryman, 1984; Cipolla & De Lillo, 2004; Olsen & Morgan, 2005), rather than on the consequences of the extension of a culture of quantification into everyday life. There are some exceptions: Mackenzie (2014) draws from a sociology of algorithms in order to explain how mathematical models shape markets; under a more ethnomethodological perspective, Suchman (2011) has investigated how instruments have material effects in the construction of scientific facts, while Mackenzie (2013) has analysed the practices by which synthetic biology constructs its legitimisation in society. From a more classic sociological stance, in his theory of communicative action, Habermas (1985) warned against the progressive colonisation of the lifeworld by the system and its instrumental rationality – yet he did not explicitly investigate quantification as a tool of instrumental rationality.

It may be that this lack of interest in quantification is due to the fact that 'In a world saturated with numbers, it is easy to take the work of quantification for granted' (Espeland & Stevens, 2008, p. 411) and that 'Counting may seem like a simple act, but doing it on a large scale requires well-funded bureaucracies with highly trained administrators' (Espeland & Stevens, 2008, p. 411). The lack of attention to the impact of quantification on everyday life has a historical dimension. The development of technology means that quantification no longer requires the support of a large bureaucracy. In contemporary society, individuals can organise their domestic activities, even their sexual lives (Lupton, 2014b), using the same principles and methodologies of large-scale commercial organisations. Technology such as smartphones enables individuals to undertake intensive self-tracking. Individuals can collect and store an enormous amount of life data, such as the number of steps they take each day, time spent in rapid eye movement (REM) sleep or the miles they run. Individuals can also track their own heart rate, body temperature, blood sugar, menstruation cycle and caloric intake. In fact, individuals can record a wide range of everyday activities, form the money they spend, the drinks they drink to the number of cigarettes they smoke. Through the construction of 'personal analytics', individuals can also bring fine-grained statistical analysis to bear on the data they collect and develop precise graphical representations. Among the visualisation types, the most common are line charts, followed by bar charts and calendars (Choe, Lee, Bongshin, & Kientz, 2014). In short, digital quantification and self-tracking aim to reconnect what Weber argued modernity had separated. For Weber:

the modern rational organization of the capitalistic enterprise would not have been possible without two other important factors in its development: the separation of business from the household, which completely dominates modern economic life, and closely connected with it, rational book-keeping. (Weber, 1992, p. 35)

Self-tracking re-establishes the link between the private household and the public sphere of business creating the 'quantified self', a concept first identified by Gary Wolf and Kevin Kelly, two editors from *Wired* magazine in 2008 (Wolf, 2010). Wolf and Kelly created a site, www.quantifiedself.com, on which people fond of self-tracking can exchange information, discuss their achievements and reflect on the effectiveness of such tracking for changing one's habits. The site has acted as a hub for an impressive number of social activities. There are more than 100 'quantified selfer' associations spread all over the world, which hold workshops every week and have an annual conference. The slogan of the site is revealing: 'self-knowledge through numbers' (see the site The Quantified Self, http://quantifiedself.com/2011/03/what-is-the-quatified-self/). Wolf described the main characteristics of the 'philosophy' of quantified selfers in a (now) famous article in the *New York Times* (2010). Its title is particularly appropriate: *The Data-Driven Life*. Wolf stressed the importance of collecting data related to our everyday life activities. He claimed that if individuals collect detailed information on themselves, as it is done by the R&D departments of big corporations, they could become more conscious of their errors, improve their habits and be more productive. In short, quantification would allow individuals to become better human beings. Hence, for many quantified selfers, self-tracking is a tool of human enhancement (Maturo, 2012).

The strong emphasis 'on numbers in the discourse and technologies associated with digital self-tracking' (Lupton, 2015, p. 7) is especially interesting. According to Wolf (2010), individuals tolerate this 'dry and mechanical' kind of knowledge because the results can be so powerful. Wolf argued that:

Numbering things allows tests, comparisons, experiments. Numbers make problems less resonant emotionally but more tractable intellectually. In science, in business and in the more reasonable sectors of government, numbers have won fair and square. (Wolf, 2010, p. 2)

Lupton (2014a) also observed that numbers render subjective experiences apparently objective. The body can be represented mathematically as a set of values, numbers and algorithms, which seem to be easily comparable across individuals.

Furthermore, this way of representing (and knowing) the body can easily be shared on social networks, shifting these previously private elements into the public sphere (Lupton, 2012). According to van Manen, social networks have been encouraging 'the privatization of the public and the publicization of the private' (Van Manen, 2010, p. 1024). Also, charming graphs and bright histograms make the quantifications appear more real and true. Indeed, visualisation is at the core of the scientific-like discourse constructed by these apps. This is particularly evident in healthcare and medicine, where magnetic resonance imaging has moved from being a valuable diagnostic tool to being an author-itative source of knowledge (Joyce, 2008) so that the primary diagnostic tool is no longer 'touch' but has become 'sight'.

Apps can be seen as 'technologies of the self' (Foucault, 1977) that shape a body which is increasingly healthy and productive. This 'disciplined' body emerges as a result of adherence to a specific regime made up of targets, rewards and punishments. Yet, the punishment is not a 'pastoral' one (one inflicted by the good shepherd), nor is it a juridical one. It is more similar to a missed bonus in a video game or losing points in a game we play on our smart phones. Indeed, one of the main features of the self-tracking experience is gamification.

The gamification of health

Gamification can be viewed as a process by which non-game activities are represented in a game-like form (Morford, Witts, & Killingsworth, 2014). Some researchers use the term ludification, which is a broader concept incorporating gamification. According to Lupton and Thomas, ludification:

> is used in the academic literature on gaming... to refer to elements of games reading into other aspects beyond leisure pursuits. (Lupton & Thomas, 2015, p.1)

Gamification has been used extensively in education programmes to promote improved learning motivation and outcomes. Currently, gamification is considered one of the most innovative and promising marketing tools (McGonigal, 2011). The idea of a reward is at the core of gamification practices, framing behavioural change in terms of points gained, levels achieved, places on leader boards, badges received and other similar markers in order to encourage users (Nichols, 2015, p. 1). According to McGonigal (2011), thanks to gamification, we will soon be able to solve the biggest problems of the world, such as cancer and climate change:

> new participation platforms and collaboration environments are making it possible for anyone to help invent the future, just by playing a game. (McGonigal, 2011, p. 15)

It is hard to deny that games play a cognitive function. According to many scholars, games and play allow people, not only children but also adults, to learn important aspects of the world (Erikson, 1963; Freud, 1920; Mead, 1934). In apps, gamification serves to support people in pursuing goals and improve performances: running faster, eating healthier and quitting smoking. The apps involve a high level of self-survcillance with incentivisation and pleasure rather than risk and fear shaping desired behaviours (Whitson, 2013, p. 167). Gamification has a perlocutionary function: it allows us to not only know things but to do them (Austin, 1962). There are aspects of gamification in most health apps. In this article, we use an extended conception of gamification and we argue that there can be varying degrees of gamification. For instance, a high level of gamification is present in the app *Streak for the Cash*. This app includes the following statement:

> Think you know your sports team? Then name your predictions for each game and make sure you get the longest winning streak of the month. The longest winning streak for a team or a player will win a monthly grand prize of $50,000.

On the other hand, there are running apps that do not appear to include any elements of gamification. However, Whitson noted that most running apps include the 'encouraging simulated voice' (2013, p. 171) designed to assist the runner, and this can be seen as a form of gamification. Whitson noted that gamification is more obvious in some apps such as *Nike+*, which has the facility to set:

challenges and goals, both short term and long term, and beating the shadow data of my past selves. As my total running distance accumulates, I earn rewards such as congratulation messages (...) and certificates of achievement. (Whitson, 2013, p. 171)

An interesting example of the gamification of health is the app *Zombies, Run!*. Users run while listening to a narrative which portrays them as a crucial member of a group of survivors of the zombie apocalypse. Periodically, they are told that they are being chased by zombies and running faster will save them and other potential victims. The app's description comments, 'and if you want a serious workout, turn on thrilling zombie chases that force you to speed up to escape the hordes!'.

According to Cummings, Goodman, Nonamaker and Golson (2013), the Generation Y (or Millennials, individuals born in the decade before the Millennium, currently aged between 18 and 27) market is particularly attractive for health-care organisations as they represent the largest population cohort the USA has ever seen. This generation is socialised to digital consumption (Secondulfo, 2014); it is the healthiest cohort and thereby least costly group to insure. Most importantly, 'they grew up with gaming and have grown accustomed to interacting with businesses through custom apps and game-based interfaces' (Cummings et al., 2013, p. 2).

The language of risk and critical theories on obesity

There are number of different possible approaches to risk theory, including the realist perspective, the Foucauldian approach and a perspective that tries to integrate rationality with emotions. The realist perspective, 'which dominates in cognitive science and medical and public health approaches to risk', treats risks as 'objective pre-existing entities' (Lupton, 2014d, p. 1). Following this approach, risk can be considered as a probability of a negative outcome or event that can be avoided by preventive action, or at least, if a preventive action is taken, the negative event is less likely to occur (The Royal Society, 1992). This approach is underpinned by calculation, quantification and rationality (Maturo, 2004). As Zinn noted (2008), those using rational strategies to manage risk and uncertainty seek to identify the best course of action by weighting pros and cons and by calculation. In this approach, experts are seen as having access to superior scientific knowledge, whereas lay people rely on inferior sources such as 'folk wisdom' or common sense (2008). Yet, from the Foucauldian perspective, this reliance on experts and their expertise is a form of power and repression, as Lupton observed:

Expert knowledges are central to neo-liberal government, providing the guidelines whereby citizens are assessed, compared against norms and rendered productive. (Lupton, 1999, p. 13)

As expert knowledge is embedded in apps through the design process, individuals using these apps will process information about their activities and their environments through the medium of these expert systems and the rationality underpinning them.

However, both Zinn (2008) and Lupton (2013c) have argued that while rational rail management is one way of dealing with future uncertainty, it is not the only one or even the best. They argue that various other approaches grounded in feeling or emotion as much as reason are used by non-experts. Zinn (2008) used the term 'in-between strategies' to refer to strategies that may have a rational element but also draw on feeling and emotions such as trust. As Szompka (2000) has argued, trust has a cognitive and an emotional component. In apps, gamification can play a role by enhancing users' optimism and motivation while they undertake burdensome activities. In this way, gamification can complement quantification in enabling app users deal with uncertain situations.

When individuals self-track, they can produce large amounts of data, personal analytics, which can serve as the basis for taking decisions. Health apps can foster health literacy and knowledge about health risks by providing users with a large amount of information about their physiology. In some cases, apps will calculate the degree of risk associated with specific behaviours. For example, the app *Life Clock* will suggest (among other advices) that its user should get out and do some walking in order to add 20 minutes to his or her life expectancy. The makers of this app appropriately claim that the 'Life Clock app uses data to let you know when the things you do affect your life expectancy' (retrieved from http://thelifeclockapp.com).

The voluminous data that app users can collect enable them to make sophisticated calculations about the consequences of selecting specific means over others; the support they receive from their 'friends' on social media while sharing results and progresses enhances their motivation for pursuing the goals. In this rationalistic framework, it is easy 'to characterize risky behaviour as non-rational and to label those who undertake such unnecessary risky actions as "irresponsible"' (Hadis, 2014, p. 466). As it is evident from research on medicalisation (Barker, 2010; Jutel & Lupton, 2015), everyone living in contemporary society can provide themselves with a self-diagnosis of some health risks. The 'last well person' is absent (Hadler, 2004). But health apps provide a way of reducing such uncertainties. In the neo-liberal vision of modern society, being healthy is a matter of personal choice, motivation and responsibility (Conrad, 2007). This vision underlays a lot of the mass media's representation of obesity and is supported by numerous epidemiological studies.

The 'obesity epidemic' has become a dominant frame for obesity in the mass media, political discourse and expert statements. In the media and in scientific literature, the obesity epidemic has been a growing fear in the last 30 years (Kwan & Trautner, 2011).

The moral panic that characterises the debate on obesity is transmitted to the people themselves. Fat bodies are seen as evidence of a person's lack of restraint, weak moral attitude and a threat to the equilibrium of the community of which she is a member (Kwan & Trautner, 2011). In this context, the entire society becomes interested in disciplining those bodies which do not conform to the right mould, with no boundaries to the limits of thinness. The refusal to adhere to the mainstream image of obesity by adopting healthy behaviours is considered 'as "irrational" and "emotional", as "defiance", "apathy" or "helpness"' (Lupton, 2014d, p. 41). It is likely that the strong emphasis that apps place on the possibility of motivational changes and personal responsibility reinforces this biomedical and neo-liberal vision of obesity. Indeed, the possibility of sharing one's progress and of auto-mutual help among the community increases motivation. The apps seem to have the potential to transform 'apathetic postponers' into 'endeavourers', giving new meaning to the expressions coined by Lupton. In this context, the disciplinary path promised by the apps invites the individual to change and to become a better person, while a deviation of too many pounds is seen as a 'choice' made by a gluttonous and lazy person.

Diet apps can be seen as expert systems that allow individuals to manage the risks of unhealthy behaviours connected to eating. In this paper, we aim to understand how quantification allows users, at least potentially, to act as experts and take eating decisions based on 'scientific' knowledge, that is, histograms and graphs summarising past records of individual eating habits. Along with quantification (the cognitive side of risk management), gamification (the emotional side of risk analysis) will be taken into account.

Gamification, part of the 'in-between strategy' of apps (Zinn, 2008), enhances motivation, which is necessary to cope with risky situations.

Methodology

In this article, we draw on a study which we undertook of 'diet apps' in 2015. Our study was based on the premise that apps are sociocultural artefacts (Lupton, 2014c) and that their design reflects norms circulating in the social settings in which they are designed, manufactured and marketed. We used content analysis to study these diet apps. According to Barker, the aim of content analysis is 'to explore the relationship between discourse and the social construction of reality, or how discourse presents particular ideas that become dominant or taken-for granted'(Barker, 2010, p. 170). In the realm of apps, this approach has been applied by Lutpon and Jutel:

> Examining the words used in the app titles and descriptions on the stores and the images used, including the logo and screenshots employed to illustrate what the app offers potential users, is a way of identifying the tacit assumptions that underpin them and their truth and authority claims. (Lupton & Jutel, 2015, p. 128)

Following Lupton's approach to this analysis (2014b), we started by searching for free apps that included the term 'diet' in the category of Health & Fitness at the Google Play store. We sampled the first 20 free apps that appeared in the search. We included app descriptions provided by the developers, comments about the selected apps in online forums and user reviews in our analysis. In addition, we downloaded and studied the 20 apps for 3 weeks. Using these data, we constructed a framework of diet apps identifying seven distinctive types or categories of diet app and categorised each app in our sample in terms of whether the characteristic was present or absent.

The categories were:

- diet as a whole (reducing food and exercising)
- diet as reducing food
- food selection
  - - user-selected food
  - - app-selected food
- Diet as exercising
  - - user-selected exercises
  - - app-selected exercises
- Body mass index (BMI)
- food nutritional chart
- awards/app support
- social support/sharing results

As for the other qualitative methodologies, content analysis is deemed to lack methodological rigour. Some scholars have suggested, with explicit reference to web-based research, that content analysis may not be comparable across researchers and in some cases may be ad hoc. Moreover, the features of the web amplify the main critics of frail 'robustness' of content analysis, that is, the lack of representativeness and reproducibleness of the sample (Herring, 2010). On the other hand, this kind of analysis leads to unexpected discoveries. Specifically in the case of content analysis on the web, some methodological innovations can be achieved and 'innovation is a vital process in the evolution of any research paradigm; without it, the paradigm would stagnate' (2010, p. 244).

Findings

As can be seen in Table 1, the diet apps varied in their functions. The main information users required in these apps included weight, goal weight (or number of kilos or pounds they plan to lose in a week), height, age and sex. Many apps also asked the user to choose the kind and the frequency of physical activity in which they typically engaged. One app also asked for the user's salary. Most of the algorithms used by these apps provided a diet plan even when the planned goals were potentially harmful. For instance, it is possible to specify a diet that will allow the user to reach 66 pounds for a female of 5 feet and 8 inches height (BMI = 13.4). The apps warn users that they are underweight, but the diet is still provided.

In our analysis, we focused on those apps which presented the most intense and involving features. The degree of involvement is calculated on the following dimensions: awards and app support (such as reminders, motivational messages from the app, avatar support) and social support/sharing (participation on platforms, sharing on social networks) (see Table 1). There are four apps that appear to be more 'social', *My Diet Coach – Weight Loss, Calorie Counter/My Fitness Pal, Diet Point – Weight Loss* and *Lose Weight WithoutDieting*. We discuss each below.

My Diet Coach – Weight Loss (app 1): This app helps consumers maintain motivation and stay committed to their goals. The app suggests several daily challenges, such as reducing the consumption of carbonated drinks or performing 20 push-ups. The app includes customised motivational reminders to help the user to stay on track and reach their goals. Both the avatar, who represents the user herself/himself, and the selfies taken before and during the diet provide the user with feedback on their progress achievements and encourage the consumer to have a healthy lifestyle (such as, be more active, cook healthy food, avoid snacking in front of the TV). If the user follows the app's guidance, he or she will receive virtual clothing and accessories for their avatar to wear in the app: the achievement of goals is rewarded through online shopping. The app also provides very practical suggestions for sticking to the diet, such as parking further away from the user's destination. It also sends reminder messages, for example, remember to drink a lot of water. Some important features are only available in the Pro version which you must pay for. These features include a 'chart' that allows the user to record 'your weight and body measurement' and the 'food craving panic button', which the app refers to as a feature 'described by our customers as a life saver'.

Calorie Counter/My Fitness Pal (app 2): According to Google Play, this is the most popular app in the Health & Fitness category. When individuals start to use it, they enter their personal details and weight goal. If the app calculates that their BMI is in the underweight category and their goal is to reduce weight, then the app sends a warning message that strongly advises the user to modify their goal. However, the user can ignore this message (even if the underweight BMI remains in the user's account information). This app focuses primarily on tracking calories consumed by the user, based on a database of more than 5 million foods. In a user-friendly, two-dimensional, graph the app displays the data about food consumption that the user has previously entered. The app also prompts the user to start losing weight with friends by connecting with them on the app's embedded social network or inviting them to join. The app encourages such

Table 1. Categorisation of weight loss apps.

	(1) Diet as a whole	(2) Diet as reducing food	(2a) User-selected food	(2b) App-selected food	(3) Diet as exercising	(3a) User-selected exercises	(3b) App-selected exercises	(4) Body mass index (BMI)	(5) Food nutritional chart	(6) Awards & app support	(7) Social support/ sharing results
(1) My Diet Coach – Weigh Loss	X		x			x		x	x	x	x
(2) Calorie Counter/ My Fitness Pal	X		x			x		x	x	x	x
(3) Diet Point – Weight Loss	X			x	x			x	x	x	x
(4) Diet Plan – 7 Days		x		x					x	x	
(5) My Diet Calories	X	x	x			x		x	x		
(6) Calories Counter	X	x	x			x		x	x		x
(7) Diet Plan	X	x	x	x	x	x		x	x		
(8) Water Diet							x				
(9) Diet Diary		x	x					x			
(10) The 90 Days Diet		x		x				x	x	x	
(11) Eat Fit		x		x				x	x		x
(12) Guidelines for Healthy Diet		x		x				x	x		
(13) Lose Weight Without Dieting	X	x	x	x	x	x		x	x	x	x
(14) Weight Loss Diet Plan		x		x					x		
(15) Japanese Diet		x		x					x		
(16) Body Building Diet		x		x					x		x
(17) Diet Planner	X		x			x		x	x		
(18) Blood Group Diet		x	x								
(19) 7 Days – Stretch & Yoga Diet					x		x				
(20) Atkins Diet Malay		x	x						x		

From the first 20 apps, the following were excluded for different reasons: Diet Pembakaran (not in English); Woman's Diary (irrelevant); and Fat Burning Diet (it is practically a commercial app).

networking by posting messages to the user such as: 'People who add friends lose weight twice more'. It is interesting to note that in the Italian version of the app, this 'community' dimension is very active. We examined some of the Italian postings and found they focused on getting information about diet plus mutual support. Those posting messages often use biomedical language and seem to have a solid knowledge about diets, calories intake, pills and integrators. However, the large majority of the posts stressed the importance of a natural way of eating, without using medical products. It is interesting to notice that many members of the online community used the app to stay in a good shape and not to lose weight. The pictures that individuals posted portrayed healthy people with beautiful bodies. Some are pictured in sexy poses: in bathing suits or tight gym pants. It was clear that the online forum had a life of its own, moving beyond dieting issues. Active online participants moved beyond diet issues to discuss other topics such as where they lived or what they did for a living.

Diet Point – Weight Loss (app 3): This app allowed the users to consult several diet plans. Each diet plan could be followed based on the weight in kilograms or pounds that the user wanted to lose in a specified period of time. The app communicated with the user via the avatar, known as Damian, the Founder of Diet Point, who sent the motivational reminders. There was a wide range of forums in which users could communicate with other users who wanted to discuss weight loss, healthy recipes or eating disorders. The app sent reminders to help users maintain motivation, as well as linking them to the encouragement provided by other users in community forums. The forum was large and had many sub-forums. Often the topics which users discussed in the forums were not related to diet, for example, one sub-forum was called 'What song best describes you?'. Even in forums explicitly focused on diet such as the 'Weight Loss Diary', participants often go off-topic. However, the app placed strong emphasis on proper hydration, considering that all the proposed diets encouraged the users to drink at least eight glasses of water at work and produced sound alerts as a reminder. The app invited all users to purchase (for US$ 24) Ulla: a plastic device that could be placed on a water bottle to remind the user to drink.

Lose Weight Without Dieting (app 4): This is an 'easy to use calorie counter'. This app encouraged users to track their food consumption on a daily basis. It was based on an electronic diary in which users wrote physical and sexual activities, in addition to recording the food they had eaten. The app had a female avatar, vaguely eroticised, who provided users with encouragement and motivation. The app's motivational support was mainly based on 'SOS tips' and the avatar suggested several ways to improve the user's healthy lifestyle. If users filled in all the information about their daily life, they would win a 'bonus' to enter the next level of the in-app game. The visual design of the app was constructed in order to motivate the users to reach their planned goals. There were avatars that provide assistance and advice, for example, if the user was experiencing cravings or was tempted to eat something outside of the approved diet, an avatar would provide encouragement to stay on track. In some cases, the user's own avatar, which represented the user inside the game of the app, became thinner as the user reported weight loss. Users started as beginners, then they could move onto novices, and so on. The final level of the gamification stated: 'you are the best one in maintaining a healthy lifestyle. Take your crown, you are a champion!' If the consumer achieved the final level, the upgrade version was free of charge. The app site described this upgrade in the following way:

Along with all of these tips, tricks, and constant guidance for healthier weight loss, you also get bonuses (pearls) for frequent use of our calorie counter! These pearls will give you a discount for purchasing the ad-free version of the app! Also, if you get enough pearls, you can even remove the ad banners for free!

It is interesting to note how one element of the prize was the removal of the ads. It is almost a confession on the part of the app itself of the uselessness and annoyingness of the app's commercial side – the basis for the existence of the app itself.

Comparison of the apps: All four apps contained elements of gamification. The four apps we focused on are more 'social' than the others in our sample. These apps pushed the user to update her data regularly and to share the obtained results with friends on social networks or on the forums with participants who are trying to achieve the same goal.

The use of app support and social support was incentivised through 'awards'. Users tracked calorie intake and physical exertion, and, at any moment, the app could tell them how many calories are left in their daily dietary allocation, the amount of calories the user was 'allowed' to consume during the rest of the day (apps 2 and 3). Apps also allowed users to track their physical activity and exercise, and then calculate their approximate calorie burn. One of the apps we examined even asked users to record the number of minutes spent in sexual activity. The algorithm then converted the time spent in sexual activity into calories burned. Moreover, these apps encouraged users to record their feelings and comment on their experiences, which could be shared with the online community. The two apps that focus on diet coaching (app 1 and app 4) were more gamified than the others: the apps' avatars will congratulate users when they reach their daily goals. Users 'had to' keep their word with the app avatar – if they failed to do so, they received disapproving messages or lost points within the app. To keep users on track, apps sent reminders, messages and grant symbolic rewards such as virtual badges or points. These apps attempted to make their communications 'warmer' and more engaging. Faced with the gamified and increasingly realistic context of this digital weight loss scenario, the social determinants of health tend to disappear from view. The digital frame tends to reinforce the idea that the only reason why people do not lose weight is their motivation or their personal failure to follow through on their behavioural changes. Users of apps tend to have the status of consumers rather than patients (Setiffi, 2014). The apps and their avatars are designed to become a part of the everyday life of users, loosening and blurring the borders between online and offline existence.

Discussion

Our analysis of these four social dieting apps showed that they use a combination of approaches, part rational and part emotional, to 'enable' users deal with the risks of obesity. The apps use quantification, generated by self-tracking, data analysis and graphic layout to provide the 'rational' component of dietary control. Alongside such quantification, gamification provides the emotional support needed to maintain motivation and continue with the diet. In this sense, it is worth underlining the validity of both the 'emotion–risk assemblage' theory (Lupton, 2013c) and the 'in-between strategy' proposed by Zinn (2008). Participating in the forums as well can be interpreted within the approaches proposed by Lupton (2013c) and Zinn (2008), that is, a rational use of a resource that fosters positive emotions, eventually aimed at keeping on diet.

Diet apps provide a representation of a user that is at once atomistically insulated from other individuals while being widely socially connected through a potential network of app users. The insulation of diet app users underpins the bracketing out of the social determinants of health as noted by Lupton (2015), despite the evidence that conditions such as obesity are known to be strongly influenced by social conditions. As Link and Phelan (2010) have demonstrated, health status – and therefore one's physical condition – is heavily conditioned by education, income and living conditions. The chances individuals have to engage in a healthy life vary according to social and economic circumstances (Pickett & Wilkinson, 2011). The individualistic view underlying diet apps depoliticises the role of the state, which reduces the responsibilities of the state for the health of its citizens (Barker, 2010). Apps foster a neo-liberal ideology that implicitly stigmatises people who are not capable of meeting the standard definition of 'healthy' (Morozov, 2013). There are agreements between health maintenance organisations and employers in order to reduce the cost of the health insurance for employees who agree to disclose their self-tracking data on physical activities. While it is currently just an individual option, after some time, it could easily develop into a social obligation. If this happens, then it is not clear how those who refuse to take part will be treated. Moreover, this loosening of the borders of personal privacy can also expand the health inequality gap. As Morozov has pointed out:

> if you are well and well-off, self-monitoring will only make things better for you. If you are none of these things, the personal prospectus could make your life much more difficult, with higher insurance premiums, fewer discounts and limited employment prospects. (Morozov, 2013, p. 240)

The typical diet app user is also likely to be a member of an online community which engages in mutual support. Often, the diet app user has the opportunity to be in touch with other diet app users who are trying to lose weight through apps and these online communities. These groups of 'partial patients' fit into Rabinow's biosociality:

> In the future, the new genetics will cease to be a biological metaphor for modern society and will become instead a circulation network of identity terms and restriction loci, around which and through which a truly new type of autoproduction will emerge, which I call 'biosociality'. (Rabinow, 1996, p. 99)

Yet in the case of diet apps, we are dealing with groups that gather together not on the basis of genetic traits but physical ones. Moreover, the digital biosocialities emerging from apps have blurred and made borders mobile, though they can be effective for the pursuit of (individual) goals. Therefore, digital biosocialities are not social subjectivities but more likely groups that gather together synaptically and in elusive ways.

The connection between biosociality and obesity is perhaps more pertinent in the case of the fat acceptance movements. These groups, that have a strong presence on Facebook and Tumblr, play a political role by denouncing the stigmatisation of the obese by 'normal' people. According to an Italian study (Maturo, 2014), fat acceptance movements are biosocialities opposed to social representations that equate thinness with good health. These movements deconstruct ideological discourses that connect biological aspects with ethical ones and lead to the social discrimination of some humans.

Along with the connections to other quantified selfers, apps also enable a relationship to develop between the user and the app 'itself'. The term 'itself' is worth reflecting on as sometimes the app (or part of it) is represented by an avatar, who can have either a female or masculine appearance. And the user can also represent *self as an avatar. Often the avatars have sexualised traits, encouraging users to imagine a relationship between themselves and the app itself.

Apps can be very intrusive in users' lives and demand an intense degree of interaction with the user (van Loon, Oudshoorn, & Bal, 2014); they send reminders, motivational prompts and congratulations for attained goals, among other communications. Another characteristic that should be mentioned about diet apps is their 'amorality'. These apps set virtually no limits on users' weight loss goals. With few exceptions, of the 20 apps we analysed, the diet was constructed or proposed without any considerations of possible dangers. Imagine that the user is 5 feet and 8 inches tall and weighs 88 pounds; he or she wants a regime that would results in a weight loss of 22 pounds, that is becoming seriously underweight. After entering these data, the app would propose a diet to reach the specified weight without any caveats. This is an issue national and supranational authorities could and should address to prevent harmful consequences. While the Food and Drug Administration regulates mobile medical applications (FDA 2015), it seems that there is an area of 'anarchy' for non-medical apps that can affect health.

Thus, diet apps present obesity as a risk wholly dependent on the individual's will to intervene. They tend to present dieting as a type of game. They are designed to show that the user can reduce the risk of obesity by controlling his or her diet and that treating dieting as game playing can make this easier. App descriptions regularly use the rhetoric of returning to the 'real me' (usually a *thin* real me) or starting a 'new [thin] life'. They use the methodology of cognitive psychology solutions as the basis of behaviour change. The framework embedded in the apps is that of the therapy culture in which any potential risk can be addressed and renormalised and that individuals can live under surveillance and in constant interaction with an expert system, in this case the app (Furedi, 2004). These apps contain no references to counter-narratives of obesity, such as fat acceptance. Apps present these diets using scientific terms and tools: graphs, percentages and fine-grained statistics legitimate and assert the reliability of the apps. The support for behaviour change is provided by the sharing culture of social networks. There is no place for any social conditions that can be connected to health such as inequalities, poverty or social stratification, features that can hardly be integrated into a 'gamified' life.

The self of the quantified self is represented by a series of percentages, histograms and measurements whose meaning is constructed through the comparison with other participants in the same programme and in relation to the numerical goals reached. The forums legitimise and support this kind of self based on graphs and numbers. Indeed, numbers become a medium and a lingua franca to start a conversation between people who do not have much in common – perhaps only the goal of losing weight. Therefore, the numbers become a strong excuse to establish an emotional relationship, which is something very distant from the dryness and coldness of measurement, but at the same time functional to this neo-liberal view of world. Also in this case, we can suggest that these forums resemble elusive biosocialities that provide mutual support to their members for partial goals and a limited amount of time: the strength of weak connections.

Conclusion

In contemporary society, through smartphones, individuals can engage in elaborate data collection and analysis, which in the past only big enterprises and large bureaucracies could afford the R&D departments necessary to do so. Self-tracking is an opportunity for potentially everyone. The ability to quantify oneself invites individuals to become self-entrepreneurs that optimise their performance. Users can apply sophisticated software programs to themselves and their bodies as if they were big organisations. Through the commensuration and quantification of their personal analytics, users are invited to run themselves through strategic planning and marketing. Today, we can organise our diet as if it were a business and therefore manage it through a rational, digital form of book-keeping. This rational record-keeping and scientific approach to life is not limited to dieting – it can be implemented on yoga, meditation and sex, to name a few (Lupton, 2014b). There are apps for virtually any human activity. The quantified self mentality is suggestive of a sort of Fordism, on an individual scale and not tied to the factory, or better, a reframing of the individual as an individual factory. This is a pleasurable Fordism for users, given the appealing designs of apps and their increasing gamification which renders such tracking into a form of play. As said, the design and the functions of the apps are connected to an idea of a subject that is functional to neo-liberal economy. Also, the practices that occur in the forums legitimise this configuration. The self of the quantified self brings to life the ideal self of economic textbooks, that is, the rational actor who makes choices to maximise his or her utility on the basis of solid information.

Our analysis of diet apps seems to validate the hypothesis that users' risk management is based on a mixed method combining quantification and gamification, which correspond to, respectively, rationality and emotions. In other words, quantification – which includes self-tracking, data analysis and graphic layout – provides the 'rational' basis for following dietary regimes, while gamification provides the emotional support to sustain motivation and keep on with the diet. Therefore, it is appropriate to stress the validity of the 'emotion–risk assemblage' theory (Lupton, 2013c) and the 'in-between strategy' (Zinn, 2008). Also, taking part in forums can be interpreted as a rational use of a resource that fosters positive emotions, which is very useful if one wants to follow a diet plan. Therefore, the two similar perspectives proposed by Lupton (2013a) and Zinn (2008), which reintegrate emotions in risk management, are applicable to the analysis of apps and digital devices for self-tracking.

The potential applications of m-health are enormous (European Commission, 2014). In this article, we have restricted our analysis to motivational apps for weight loss. On the basis of our research, we think that a series of risks should be taken into consideration:

- The reductionist conception that obesity is an individual problem and that becoming thinner depends basically on individual motivation shifts focus away from important social conditions which are known to deeply impact health conditions.
- Any connection with the social and political dimensions of obesity is downplayed, which limits the kinds of solutions we may consider.
- There are few warnings or safety restrictions aimed at the people who choose to follow a diet using an app: this may serve to exacerbate conditions such as anorexia nervosa and encourage disordered behaviour in all populations. National and supranational authorities should intervene, despite the recognised law lag that plagues institutional responses to Internet innovation, given the astonishing number of apps available to users.
- There are risks of discrimination between people who choose to share their self-tracking data and people who do not – especially in the area of health coverage.

More research should be done to integrate the astonishing possibilities opened by the quantification of life and an approach based on social determinants of health. There is no app for ensuring social justice.

Acknowledgements

While this article is the result of several discussions between the authors, Francesca Setiffi wrote the sections 'The Gamification of Health', 'Methodology' and 'Findings' and Antonio Maturo wrote the remainder of the article. The reviewers provided us with invaluable help with their comments and remarks.

Disclosure statement

No potential conflict of interest was reported by the authors.

References

Austin, J. L. (1962). *How to do things with words*. London: Oxford University Press.
Barker, K. K. (2010). The social construction of illness: Medicalization and contested illness. In C. Bird, P. Conrad, A. Freemont, & S. Timmermans (Eds.), *Handbook of medical sociology* (pp. 147–162). Nashville: Vanderbilt U.P.
Bryman, A. (1984). The debate about qualitative and quantitative research. A question of methods or epistemology. *The British Journal of Sociology*, *35*(1), 75–92. doi:10.2307/590553
Choe, E. K., Lee, N. B., Bongshin, L., & Kientz, J. A. (2014). *Understanding quantified-selfers' practices in collecting and exploring personal data*. Proceedings ACM Human Factors in Computing Systems, 1143–1152. doi:10.1145/2556288.2557372
Cipolla, C., & De Lillo, A. (Eds.). (2004). *Il sociologo e le sirene. La sfida dei metodi qualitativi* [The Sociologist and the Sirens. The Challenge of Qualitative Methods]. Milano: FrancoAngeli Editore.
Conrad, P. (2007). *The medicalization of society: On the transformation of human conditions into treatable disorders*. Baltimore: Johns Hopkins University Press.
Cummings, P., Goodman, D., Nonamaker, L., & Golson, M. (2013). *Gaming to engage the healthcare consumer* (White paper: ICF International, 1-7). Retrieved from http://www.icfi.com/insights/white-papers/2013/gaming-to-engage-healthcare-consumer
Erikson, E. H. (1963). *Childhood and Society*. New York, NY: Norton.
Espeland, W. N., & Stevens, M. L. (2008). A sociology of quantification. *European Journal of Sociology*, *49*(3), 401–436. doi:10.1017/S0003975609000150
European Commission. (2014). *Green paper on mobile health* (mHealth) (Paper No. 219). Retrieved from European Commission - Digital Agenda for Europe: http://ec.europa.eu/digital-agenda/en/news/green-paper-mobile-health-mhealth
Flegal, K. M., Graubard, B. I., Williamson, D. F., & Gail, M. H. (2005). Excess deaths associated with underweight, overweight, and obesity. *The Journal of the American Sociological Association*, *93*(15), 1861–1867. doi:10.1001/jama.293.15.1861
Food and Drug Administration. (2015), Mobile medical applications. Guidance for Industry and Food and Drug Administration Staff, Document issued on February 9, 2015. Retrieved from http://www.fda.gov/downloads/MedicalDevices/DeviceRegulationandGuidance/GuidanceDocuments/UCM263366.pdf
Foucault, M. (1977). *Discipline and punish: The birth of the prison*. New York, NY: Pantheon.
Freud, S. (1920). *On metaphyschology*. London: Penguin Books.
Furedi, F. (2004). *Therapy culture*. London: Routledge.
Guseva, A. (2013). *Consumerism in health care*. Oxford: The Wiley-Blackwell Encyclopaedia of Health, Illness, Behavior, and Society, Wiley-Blackwell.
Habermas, J. (1985). *The theory of communicative action*. Boston, MA: Beacon Press.
Hadis, B. F. (2014). Risk, social protection and trust amidst cuts in welfare spending. *Health, Risk & Society*, *16*(5), 459–480. doi:10.1080/13698575.2014.936832
Hadler, N. M. (2004). *The last well person: How to stay well despite the health-care system*. Montreal: McGill-Queen's University Press.

Herring, S. C. (2010). Web content analysis: Expanding the paradigm. In J. Hunsinger, L. Klastrup, & M. Allen (Eds.), *International handbook of internet research* (pp. 233–249). New York, NY: Springer.

Joyce, K. A. (2008). *Magnetic appeal. MRI and the Myth of transparency*. Ithaca: Cornell University Press.

Jutel, A., & Lupton, D. (2015). Digitizing diagnosis: A review of mobile applications in the diagnostic process. *Diagnosis*, 1–8. doi:10.1515/dx-2014-0068

Kwan, S., & Trautner, M. N. (2011). Weighty concerns. *Contexts*, *10*(2), 52–57. doi:10.1177/1536504211408907

Light, D., & Maturo, A. (2015). *Good pharma. The public-health model of the Mario Negri Institute*. New York, NY: Palgrave.

Link, B., & Phelan, J. (2010). Social conditions as fundamental causes of health inequalities. In C. Bird, P. Conrad, A. Freemont, & S. Timmermans (Eds.), *Handbook of medical sociology* (pp. 3–17). Nashville: Vanderbilt University Press.

Lupton, D. (1999). *Risk*. London: Routledge.

Lupton, D. (2012). M-health and health promotion: The digital cyborg and surveillance society. *Social Theory & Health*, *10*(3), 229–244. doi:10.1057/sth.2012.6

Lupton, D. (2013a). *Risk* (2nd ed.). London: Routledge.

Lupton, D. (2013b). The digitally engaged patient: Self-monitoring and self-care in the digital health era. *Social Theory & Health*, *11*(3), 256–270. doi:10.1057/sth.2013.10

Lupton, D. (2013c). Risk and emotion: Towards an alternative theoretical perspective. *Health, Risk & Society*, *15*(8), 634–647. doi:10.1080/13698575.2013.848847

Lupton, D. (2014a). The commodification of patient opinion: The digital patient experience economy in the age of big data. *Sociology of Health & Illness*, *36*, 856–869. doi:10.1111/1467-9566.12109

Lupton, D. (2014b). Quantified sex: A critical analysis of sexual and reproductive self-tracking apps. *Culture, Health & Sexuality*, *17*(4), 440–453. doi:10.1080/13691058.2014.920528

Lupton, D. (2014c). Apps as artefacts: Towards a critical perspective on mobile health and medical apps. *Societies*, *4*(4), 606–622. doi:10.3390/soc4040606

Lupton, D. (2014d). *Risk*. The Wiley-Blackwell Encyclopaedia of Health, Illness, Behavior, and Society. Oxford: Wiley-Blackwell.

Lupton, D. (2015). *Digital sociology*. London: Routledge.

Lupton, D., & Jutel, A. (2015). 'It's like having a physician in your pocket!' A critical analysis of selfdiagnosis smartphone apps. *Social Science and Medicine*, *133*, 128–135. doi:10.1016/j.socscimed.2015.04.004

Lupton, D., & Thomas, G. M. (2015). Playing pregnancy: The ludification and gamification of expectant motherhood in smartphone apps. *M/C Journal*, *18*(5), 1–8. Retrieved from http://journal.media-culture.org.au/index.php/mcjournal/article/viewArticle/1012

Mackenzie, A. (2013). From validating to verifying: Public appeals in synthetic biology. *Science as Culture*, *22*(4), 476–496. doi:10.1080/14636778.2013.764067

Mackenzie, D. (2014, June). *A Sociology of Algorithms: High-Frequency Trading and the Shaping of Markets*. Working paper. Retrieved from http://www.sps.ed.ac.uk/__data/assets/pdf_file/0004/156298/Algorithms25.pdf

Maturo, A. (2004). Network governance as a response to risk society' dilemmas: A proposal from sociology of health. *Topoi – International Review of Philosophy*, *23*(2), 195–202. doi:10.1023/B:TOPO.0000046066.21486.82

Maturo, A. (2012). Social justice and human enhancement in today's bionic society. *Salute e Società*, *XI*(2), 15–28. Retrieved from http://www.francoangeli.it/riviste/Scheda_rivista.aspx?IDArticolo=47776

Maturo, A. (2014). Fatism, self-monitoring and the pursuit of healthiness in the time of technological solutionsim. *Italian Sociological Review*, *4*(2), 157–171. Retrieved from http://www.italiansociologicalreview.org/attachments/article/173/3%20Fatism%20SelfMonitoring%20and%20the%20Pursuit%20of%20Healthiness%20in%20the%20Time%20of%20Technological%20Solutionism_Maturo.pdf

McGonigal, J. (2011). *Reality is broken. How games are making us better and how they can change the world*. New York, NY: The Penguin Press.

Mead, G. H. (1934). *Mind, self and society*. Chicago: University of Chicago Press.

Morford, Z. H., Witts, B. N., & Killingsworth, M. P. (2014). Gamification: The intersection between behavior analysis and game design technologies. *The Behavior Analyst, 37*, 25–40. doi:10.1007/s40614-014-0006-1

Morozov, E. (2013). *To save everything, click here: Technology, solutionism, and the urge to fix problems that don't exist.* London: Penguin.

Nichols, S. (2015). A RECIPE for meaningful gamification. In T. Reiners & L. C. Wood (Eds.), *Gamification in education and business* (pp. 1-20)). Switzerland: Springer.

Olsen, W., & Morgan, J. (2005). A critical epistemology of analytical statistics: Addressing the sceptical realist. *Journal for the Theory of Social Behaviour, 35*, 255–284. doi:10.1111/j.1468-5914.2005.00279.x

Pickett, K., & Wilkinson, R. (2011). *The spirit level: Why greater equality makes societies stronger.* New York, NY: Bloomsbury.

Prochaska, J. O., & Velicer, W. F. (1997). The transtheoretical model of health behavior change. *American Journal of Health Promotion, 12*(1), 38–48. doi:10.4278/0890-1171-12.1.38

Rabinow, P. (1996). *Anthropology of Reason.* Princeton: Princeton U.P.

Ruckenstein, M. (2014). Visualized and interacted life: Personal analytics and engagements with data doubles. *Societies, 4*(1), 68–84. doi:10.3390/soc4010068

Secondulfo, D. (2014). Born to buy. The socialization of young consumers. *Italian Journal of Sociology of Education, 6*(3), 26–40. Retrieved from http://www.ijse.eu/wp-content/uploads/2014/10/2014_3_3.pdf

Setiffi, F. (2014). Becoming consumers: Socialization into the world of goods. *Italian Journal of Sociology of Education, 6*(3), 6–25. Retrieved from http://www.ijse.eu/wp-content/uploads/2014/10/2014_3_2.pdf

Suchman, L. (2011). Practice and its overflows: Reflections on order and mess, *Tecnoscienza. Italian Journal of Science and Technology, 2*(1), 21–30.

Sullivan, D. A. (2010). A social change model of the obesity epidemic. In A. Mukherjea (Ed.), *Understanding emerging epidemics: Social and political approaches* (pp. 315–342). London: Emerald.

Sztompka, P. (2000). *Trust. A sociological theory.* Cambridge: Cambridge University Press.

The Royal Society. (1992), Risk Analysis, Perception and Management. Retrieved from The Royal Society: https://royalsociety.org/topics-policy/publications/1992/risk/

Van Loon, E., Oudshoorn, N., & Bal, R. (2014). Studying design and use of healthcare technologies in interaction: The social learning perspective in a dutch quality improvement collaborative program. *Health, 6*, 1903–1918. doi:10.4236/health.2014.615223

Van Manen, M. (2010). The pedagogy of Momus technologies: Facebook, privacy and online intimacy. *Qualitative Health Research, 20*(8), 1023–1032. doi:10.1177/1049732310364990

Weber, M. (1992). *The protestant ethic and the spirit of capitalism.* New York, NY: Routledge.

Whitson, J. R. (2013). Gaming the quantified self. *Surveillance & Society, 11*(1/2), 163–172. Retrieved from http://library.queensu.ca/ojs/index.php/surveillance-and-society/article/view/gaming/0

Wolf, G. (2010, April 28). The data-driven life. *The New York Times Magazine.* Retrieved from http://www.nytimes.com/2010/05/02/magazine/02self-measurement-t.html?_r=0

Zinn, J. O. (2008). Heading into the unknown: Everyday strategies for managing risk and uncertainty. *Health, Risk & Society, 10*(5), 439–450. doi:10.1080/13698570802380891

Threats and thrills: pregnancy apps, risk and consumption

Gareth M. Thomas[a] and Deborah Lupton[b]

[a]School of Social Sciences, Cardiff University, Cardiff, UK; [b]Faculty of Arts and Design, University of Canberra, Canberra, Australia

In this article, we draw on the findings of a critical discourse analysis of pregnancy-related mobile software applications designed for smartphones ('apps') to examine how such apps configure pregnant embodiment. Drawing on a detailed analysis of all such apps available in June 2015 in the two major global app stores Google Play and Apple App Store, we discuss how such technologies (the 'threats' mode of representation) portray the pregnant body as a site of risk requiring careful self-surveillance using apps to reduce potential harm to women and particularly their foetuses. We show that the second dominant mode of representation ('thrills') constructs the pregnant body and self-tracking in more playful terms. App developers use ludification strategies and encourage the social sharing of pregnancy-related details as part of emphasising the enjoyable aspects of pregnancy. We found that both types of pregnancy-related apps endorse expectations around pregnancy behaviour that reproduce heteronormative and gendered ideals around sexuality, parenthood and consumption. These apps are socio-cultural artefacts enacting pregnant bodies as sites of both risk and pleasure. In both cases, users of the apps are encouraged to view pregnancy as an embodied mode of close monitoring and surveillance, display and performance.

Introduction

In this article, we draw on the findings of a critical discourse analysis of pregnancy-related mobile software applications designed for smartphones ('apps') to examine how such apps configure pregnant embodiment. We identify how apps portray pregnancy and foetal bodies in particular ways as well as the implications these representations have for ideas about risk and health with respect to human fertility and reproduction.

Digital apps and pregnancy

Digital technologies are playing an increasingly important role in healthcare and the communication of information about risk and health (Lupton, 2014b, 2015a, 2015b; Rich & Miah, 2014). Mobile software applications (apps) are a central technology in digital health and risk communication. There are now over 100,000 health and medical apps available for use by lay people and healthcare workers (Jahns, 2014). Apps directed at pregnancy constitute a major genre. Hundreds of apps are available that focus on pregnancy, and many of them are very popular. Yet little social research has been conducted that has attempted to address the content of such apps and how they seek to attract interest from potential users. In this article, we draw on the findings of a critical discourse analysis of all pregnancy-related apps available in June 2015 in the two major global app stores Google Play and Apple App Store. We use these data to identify the ways in which pregnant and foetal embodiment are represented in these apps, including the discourses and practices related to health and risk that they portray.

Pregnant women have employed online technologies for information and support since the Internet became available for general use. In the early years of online communication (often characterised as the Web 1.0 era), they interacted on discussion forums and sought information from pregnancy information websites and blogs (Doty & Dworkin, 2014). The diversity of media available to pregnant women has expanded since the advent of new digital media and mobile ubiquitous computing devices (or what have been described as Web 2.0 or the social web technologies). They are now able to use a range of digital media – such as websites, blogs, podcasts, YouTube and social media (Facebook, Twitter and Instagram) – and access these using mobile devices.

Pregnancy apps are among this new range of technologies available to women and their partners. Download figures from the major app stores demonstrate the high level of interest in pregnancy app among mobile device users, with the 'I'm Expecting – Pregnancy App' attracting between 1 and 5 million downloads from the Google Play store alone. Likewise, the Apple App Store's list of popular health and fitness apps in June 2015 featured several pregnancy-related apps such as 'Period Diary' (a fertility and ovulation tracker), 'My Pregnancy Today', 'Pregnancy & Baby – What to Expect' and 'Baby Names'.

Recently researchers have shown that pregnant women are using apps in significant numbers and finding them helpful sources of information and support (Declercq, Sakala, Corry, Applebaum, & Herrlich, 2013; Derbyshire & Dancey, 2013; Hearn, Miller, & Fletcher, 2013; Kraschnewski et al., 2014; Peyton, Poole, Reddy, Kraschnewski, & Chuang, 2014; Rodger et al., 2013). A large-scale survey conducted with American women who had recently given birth (Declercq et al., 2013) found that 56% of first-time mothers rated pregnancy apps as providing valuable information, as did 47% of experienced mothers. Another American study (Kraschnewski et al., 2014) involving a series of focus groups carried out with pregnant women revealed that they used online sites and apps for pregnancy information since prenatal care was not meeting their needs. Australian research (Rodger et al., 2013), drawing on qualitative interviews with pregnant women, found that many of them had downloaded a smartphone app. Researchers who conducted a survey of pregnant women at an Irish maternity hospital (O'Higgins et al., 2014) showed that 59% had used a pregnancy app. These apps were viewed as particularly important for disadvantaged women who may lack access to other educational resources.

Healthcare and public health professionals have begun to suggest that women's use of apps will influence maternity care and that they should be considered in the future planning of care provision (Hearn et al., 2013, 2014; O'Higgins et al., 2014; Robinson & Jones, 2014; Rodger et al., 2013; Tripp et al., 2014). From the perspective of midwives, for example, Robinson and Jones (2014) stress the importance of professionals acknowledging the widespread use of apps by pregnant women. They assert that apps may empower and inform women so that they take more responsibility for their health but that the quality of information offered is often dubious and may supplant professional advice.

Apps, like any other form of media, are forms of texts and sociocultural artefacts that both draw on and reproduce shared norms, ideals, knowledges and beliefs (Lupton, 2014a, 2015b; Lupton & Jutel, 2015), including those related to health and risk. They are worthy of sustained critical analysis that is able to identify these features. Health and medical app topics can suggest trends in health and medical regimes, treatments and conditions as well as methods in medical education and training. The ways in which they verbally and visually represent the human body provide insights into contemporary notions of embodiment, health, disease and risk. Thus far, however, few researchers have adopted this perspective on apps of any type. While there is a growing body of research related to the content of health and medical apps, this tends to focus on evaluating the accuracy or validity of their content rather than seeking to identify their wider social, cultural and political implications.

Despite their popularity, little comprehensive research has been conducted into the content of pregnancy-related apps, with a few important exceptions. Tripp et al. (2014) analysed 430 apps judged to be related to pregnancy and divided them into four categories: informative, interactive, tools and social media. Tripp et al. found, based on the number of reviewers per app, that the informative (non-interactive) apps were the most popular, followed by interactive apps that allowed women to upload information and customise displays. Johnson (2014) adopted a more critical approach in discussing the implications of a limited selection of apps, as well as other digital technologies, for the responsibilisation of pregnant women in the context of monitoring their own and their foetus's bodies. Finally, Lupton's (2015b) work on sexuality and reproductive self-tracking apps found there was a strongly heteronormative dimension incorporated into these apps. Female sexuality and reproductive capacities were represented as oriented towards careful self-monitoring of fertility, avoiding and facilitating conception and risk avoidance. In contrast, male sexuality was portrayed as performative and competitive.

The research we draw on in this article enables us to build on these studies by combining a comprehensive overview of pregnancy-related apps with a critical discourse analysis approach to their content. We identify how apps portray pregnancy and foetal bodies in particular ways as well as the implications these representations have for ideas about risk and health with respect to human fertility and reproduction (Coxon, 2014; Lupton, 2013).

Methods

Critical discourse analysis focuses attention on the social, cultural and political dimensions of texts, and what they reveal about tacit assumptions and power relations. Discourse is viewed as a form of social practice that is socially constitutive and shaped (Fairclough, Mulderrig, & Wodak, 2011). As we note above, apps are cultural texts and communicative agents that make certain truth claims, and their developers use carefully chosen images and discourses to represent their use and function to attract downloads. Critical discourse analysis is able to identify these tacit assumptions, norms and truth claims that such texts articulate and convey to their audiences.

Google Play and the Apple App Store are the two major platforms offering apps; they have a combined market share of 91% of apps installed on mobile phones (Seneviratne, Seneviratne, Mohapatra, & Mahanti, 2015). As of May 2015, 1.5 million apps were available to download on Google Play while 1.4 million were available on the Apple App Store (Statista, 2015b). From June 2008 to June 2015, the cumulative number of apps downloaded from the Apple App Store reached 100 billion (Statista, 2015a). We undertook a search for all pregnancy-related apps offered in these platforms in June 2015, using key terms including pregnancy, childbirth, conception, foetus/fetus and baby. After both authors agreed on the types of apps that we intended to include in our sample, the first author (Gareth Thomas) carried out the preliminary searches. These were shared with the second author (Deborah Lupton), who conducted further searches to identify apps missed in earlier searches, thus ensuring that the process was rigorous and consistent. When the inclusion of particular apps was thrown into doubt by one author, this was discussed with the other author and a decision was made about inclusion or exclusion in the sample.

As we wanted to explore the complete range of different portrayals of pregnancy for the full variety of purposes and audiences, we included all human pregnancy-related apps in our analysis, including those directed at fertility monitoring and preconception care and those that involved games and other entertainment-related pursuits. After eliminating apps listed in these searches that were clearly not related to human pregnancy, we were left with 665 apps on Google Play and 1141 on the Apple App Store for inclusion in our study (many of these apps were shared across the stores). We undertook a critical discourse analysis of the descriptions of these apps offered on the two app stores. We paid attention to the title of each app, the textual accounts of its content and use and the images that were employed, such as the logo of the app and the screenshots that were used to illustrate its content and style.

Findings

In the apps we reviewed, we noted that the vast majority of pregnancy apps could be grouped into three main categories: 'entertainment', 'pregnancy and foetal monitoring' and 'pregnancy information'. The first category, 'entertainment', included games, pregnancy test and ultrasound pranks, shopping for pregnancy-related products, quizzes to test pregnancy knowledge, gender predictors and baby name generators. The second category of apps, 'pregnancy and foetal monitoring', provided functions that encouraged women to monitor and survey the foetus and pregnant body. This included tracking weight and waist measurements, diet, water consumption, symptoms, moods, medications, cravings, appetite and energy levels. Other apps in this category allowed women to input due dates and appointments, record foetal heartbeat and movement, write journals and create scrapbooks and share ultrasound images and biometric data such as foetal movement (for example, kicks and heartbeats) with health professionals as well as friends and family members via social media. Taken together, these apps allowed for the production of a repository of personal medical information.

The third major category, 'pregnancy information', offered a range of information about pregnancy, including details about foetal development, nutrition and exercise in pregnancy and substances and behaviours that should be avoided by pregnant women in the interests of maintaining their own health and promoting the health and optimum development of their foetus. Some information apps also provided women with access to online forums in which to connect to other pregnant women (for example, to share and compare stories and experiences).

There were also several additional (separate) categories but these were much fewer in number. This included the categories of 'labour and childbirth', 'medical', 'preconception and fertility' and 'for fathers'. Labour and childbirth apps were mostly those which allowed women or their partners or both to measure and monitor contractions, but could also include those which provided relaxation techniques for labour and created a birth plan and checklist for both the birth and newborn equipment and products. A group of apps provided medical information and training for health professionals and students (including quizzes for medical exams). Whilst there were several apps available for preconception and fertility (such as giving advice about fertility and infertility, apparent pregnancy tests, ovulation and menstruation trackers), only a small number of pregnancy-related apps were explicitly directed at fathers.

In analysing our corpus of apps, we started to recognise how, across these categories, apps could be divided into two major themes: one in which pregnancy was enacted as a highly risky state in need of careful management (characterised by us as 'threats'), and one in which it was constituted as a site of pleasure, enjoyment and entertainment (or 'thrills'). While these themes may appear very different, we noted that both incorporated ideas about the importance of pregnant women tracking their bodies, and in some cases, sharing their personal data with others. We elaborate on these themes in the following sections.

Threats: pregnant and foetal bodies at risk

There are a plethora of apps allowing pregnant women to monitor their body (weight, diet, mood, etc.) and that of the foetus (growth, heartbeat, etc.), access information on health for pregnancy and childbirth, and share concerns and data with health professionals together with other pregnant women, family and friends. Such apps, we argue, frequently render the pregnant body as risky and in need of self-monitoring and surveillance. This is achieved in many different ways, from alluding to the importance of *attaining* a 'normal' or 'perfect' pregnancy to citing scientific endorsement to provide legitimacy.

This 'risk' and 'health management' discourse emerged in apps like 'Ovia Pregnancy Tracker', a popular app with 100,000–500,000 downloads on Google Play alone, which adopted a 'high-tech, personalised approach to tracking your baby's development and pregnancy week by week'. In order to 'have a healthier pregnancy', users were encouraged to gain 'immediate feedback' by using 'data science and your personal information' to track weight, sleep and symptoms (among other things) and 'deliver personal and baby development milestones' as well as 'immediate health risks'. The app encouraged women to track their weight gain, pregnancy symptoms (and receive alerts if these symptoms 'indicate a health risk'), food, fluid and vitamin intake, sleep, moods and exercise. The app provided users with the opportunity to research symptoms to determine 'is this normal for pregnancy' as well as medication and food safety. One screenshot, for instance, was headed by 'Are my symptoms normal?' accompanied by a photograph of a woman holding her bare bump and the tagline 'know when to call your doctor'. Like other apps, Ovia was advertised as allowing women to 'have a healthier pregnancy' by receiving daily updates on pregnancy and baby size/development, 'critical health alerts for pregnancy risks on analysis of your data' and over 400 articles and 'tools'.

The legitimacy of 'Ovia Pregnancy Tracker' was claimed by reference to positive user reviews and news media coverage. It included a lengthy paragraph on the 'history and science behind Ovia' (that is the use of algorithms), and the claim that it has been developed by 'Harvard scientists, pregnancy specialists and fit moms'. Claiming expertise and legitimacy by referring to a specialist's involvement in app development was a common trend we observed. Similar to Ovia, 'Pregnancy Companion by OBGYN' was described as 'the ONLY pregnancy app written and recommended by Board-certified OBGYN doctors' and as 'like having your own doctor's trusted advice (and lots of cool tools!) right at your fingertips'. Similarly, the developers of another app targeted at mothers, 'First Time Pregnancy', asserted that using the apps would 'keep you safe', especially during a first pregnancy where 'many questions and lack of information can lead to confusion or even anxiety about your own health'. This 'educational tool' was framed as being 'developed by a medical doctor with nothing but your health in mind' and a device to use 'as your personal tracker'. Screenshots of the app likewise invited users to 'get foetus details' and weekly updates, calculate due date and 'plan ahead'.

This promotion of accomplishing foetal and maternal health via apps was also enacted by 'Pregnancy Health Help and Advice Free'. Since mothers 'want to give your baby a healthy start', this app discussed 'the most important topics in pregnancy health' (for example, Caesarean, childbirth, diabetes, foetal alcohol syndrome and genetic counselling) and was directed to – as well as health professionals and students – 'lay people who just want to learn more about pregnancy health' (although with a disclaimer that it is 'for informational purposes only' and should not displace medical recommendations/professional advice). Further, the description of 'Pregnancy 41 Weeks' contained only medical information around how pregnancy begins and develops while one screenshot encouraged women to 'organise and get ready well in advance for motherhood'. This was achieved, according to the app, by taking measures 'to keep you protected' such as abstaining from alcohol and drug use as they 'may lead to serious respiratory complications, serious alcohol syndromes, birth defects and so on'.

There were also apps available for prenatal screening, high-risk pregnancies and genetic conditions. For example, 'Guide to High-Risk Pregnancy' provided women with greatly detailed medical information on 'maternal and foetal problems, ultrasound images, foetal monitor tracings and a list of worrisome conditions that can happen before or during pregnancy'. Based on a book 'Your High-Risk Pregnancy', the app had sections on diabetes, hypertension and preeclampsia, and 'normal foetal growth ultrasound measurements'. The app also contained another feature which provided women with the means to search over 4000 keywords 'to let you check out virtually any test, ultrasound or exam finding, or condition – in the doctor's office, in the ultrasound room or in the hospital'. Others apps like 'Pregnancy Risk Calculator' offered 'pregnancy risks based on certain test factors' while 'Panorama NIPT' supplied users information on how non-invasive prenatal testing for trisomies, triploidy, gene micro-deletions and monosomy X 'fits into their pregnancy journey'.

Related to this, 'Pregnancy Birth Defects' was an app which, due to 'recent medical advances' that remain unspecified, 'helps you to prevent your baby from having Down syndrome and other birth defects' as well as muscular dystrophy, Tay–Sachs disease, fragile X syndrome, Thalassemia, sickle-cell disease, cystic fibrosis and cerebral palsy. According to its description, this 'obstetrician recommended' app gave women with the opportunity to monitor foetal heartbeat, gather instructions on baby care and managing potential pregnancy problems, view images of foetal development and ensure they could 'take steps to protect your baby's health before he is born'. One such 'tip' was 'preventing' cystic fibrosis and sickle-cell anaemia by 'testing at the first visit or before conception'. Other features of the app, like many others, included a hospital appointment planner ('record your doctor's answers to your questions'), to-do list templates, a hospital bag checklist for delivery, a list of obstetrician-recommended 'newborn essentials', a personalised timeline which 'adjusts to your baby's milestones and both a weight and a contraction tracker.

Interestingly, this constellation of responsible practices directed at pregnant women was very different from the expectations inherent in the pregnancy apps that were directly targeted to prospective fathers. Although these are fewer in number, the available apps often contained 'titbits' of information rather than the vast realms offered to pregnant users (see also Johnson, 2014). As with the pregnancy apps discussed above directed at pregnant users, those for men are embedded within (hetero)normative and highly gendered ideologies assuming certain interests and capacities. One app for fathers, mPregnancy, offered advice on building furniture for and fitting out nurseries for the new infant and managing family finances, while very few, if any, apps designed for women provided similar information.

Further, pregnancy apps for men – often grounded in humour – frequently suggested that the expectant (and 'good') father would need to discipline his sexual interest in other women, offer constant reassurance to his pregnant partner that she is normal and attractive in his eyes (despite her altered physical state) and take an interest in the biometric information of their partner. In addition, fathers-to-be were framed as inherently uninterested in pregnancy and as holding little knowledge, with fatherhood depicted as 'keeping up appearances' rather than as a serious engagement with parenthood (Johnson, 2014). Whilst pregnancy apps for men were designed to be terse, matter-of-fact, humorous and simplistic (as if men did not have enough interest for large tracts of information), apps targeted at pregnant women constructed them as serious experts responsible for ensuring a 'normal' and healthy pregnancy outcome.

Thrills: the ludification of pregnant and foetal bodies

In conjunction with the many pregnancy-based apps which constructed the pregnant body as a site of risk, there was a larger collection of apps framing pregnancy as a form of entertainment and pleasure. The term 'ludification' is used in the academic literature on gaming (sometimes referred to as 'ludology') to refer to elements of games reaching into other aspects of life beyond leisure pursuits (Frissen, Lammes, De Lange, De Mul, & Raessens, 2015). This was a clear element in many pregnancy apps, including those directed at audiences other than pregnant women themselves (Lupton & Thomas, 2015). In some cases, the pregnant body itself – and the foetus within – was constituted as a consumable. Hundreds of apps allowed users to play games related to pregnancy, shop for pregnancy and baby products, predict a baby's gender, write journals, take photos, generate baby names, research baby size and compare this to inanimate objects such as fruit (such as 'Cute Fruit'), participate in quizzes, pull pregnancy 'pranks' and monitor foetal heartbeats and kicks to share with others using social media.

These apps are worthy of consideration because like the more serious apps to which we refer above, they reproduced both popular and problematic discourses around pregnancy, motherhood and fatherhood, families and the unborn. This was particularly true with respect to a significant genre of pregnancy-related apps directed at young girls. These apps positioned them as helpers, friends or medical professionals interacting with pregnant women. One app, 'Barbara Goes Shopping', has 1–5 million downloads on Google Play and involved users playing the game as Barbara's 'closest friend'. The app description began with the following:

> I've got wonderful news for you girls: our darling Barbara is expecting a baby! Barbara and Ben are so happy and excited, but yet a bit worried: they will become parents soon, and it is a great responsibility. They have already bought everything their baby will need: a stroller, loads of diapers, bottles and dummies of all kinds, pretty teddy bears, dolls and rattles and so on. But still Barbara is feeling a bit unconfident. Don't you think she needs something to cheer her up? And every girl knows that there is no better way to raise girl's spirits than a nice shopping spree!

In this statement it is clear that the happily expectant couple, Barbara and Ben, had already invested in their infant with the purchase of many products and were now ready to focus their attention on spending money to make Barbara attractive and, thus, more confident. Gamers were encouraged to visit boutiques and help Barbara purchase an outfit to 'make her feel beautiful throughout her pregnancy'. Once the game was completed, the user was notified that 'Barbara is her fashionable self again and feels prepared to welcome her baby!' The advertising image for the app was a shot of a heavily pregnant Barbara, with long blonde hair and blue eyes, wearing a pink dress and smiling as she held a blue dress (very similar in appearance to Mattel's Barbie Doll). In supplementary screenshots, Barbara – again with a pink-coloured store as a backdrop – tried on dresses, browses shoes and jewellery and experiments with different hairstyles before purchasing her goods.

This app represented the many games directed towards young girls in the market related to pregnancy that we found in the app stores. Their intended audience was clear both explicitly (that is, having the term 'girls' in the title or in the app description) and implicitly (through colours and imaging typically associated with young girls). Such games frequently asked users to either care for pregnant women or their newborn baby (or both), help pregnant women shop for clothes and food (for example, 'Lila Pregnant Shopping', 'Pregnant Mom Shopping' and 'Pregnant Mom Food Shopping'), engage in domestic cleaning (for example, 'Mother House – Cleaning Games', 'Pregnant Barbara Bath Cleaning', 'Princess Cleaning Room' and 'Pregnant Mom Washing Dishes') and give pregnant women makeovers and beautify them so that they were able to feel more confident and looked more attractive (for example, 'Pregnant Princess Beauty Salon', Pregnancy Nail Art Salon', 'Pregnant Mommy Makeover Spa' and 'Pregnancy Beauty Dress Up').

These apps portrayed the 'yummy-mummy' idealised archetype of pregnant embodiment, described by Littler (2013, p. 227–8) as a 'social type' of a mother who is 'sexually attractive and well-groomed, and who knows the importance of spending time on herself'. An archetype gaining force as it is repeated across different media, the yummy-mummy 'bodies forth' a new framing of mothers and 'espouses a girlish, high-consuming maternal ideal as a site of hyperindividualised psychological "maturity"' (Littler, 2013, p. 227). Whilst the apps described above were chiefly designed for young girls, the reproduction of gender expectations in conjunction with the idealised 'yummy-mummy' figure (such as being well-groomed) was evident. Mothers in such games were also frequently cast in gender-based fantastical, popular or fairy-tale roles including princess, mermaid, queen, fairy, nurse or celebrity, while male characters appeared beside women as princes, kings, doctors and/or supportive husbands or partners.

Other sets of apps directed at pregnant women themselves also placed emphasis on the woman's bodily appearance and/or that of the foetus. These included apps for photographing pregnancy bumps and creating time-lapse videos of transformations over time, creating 'foetal albums' of ultrasounds or for manipulating foetal ultrasounds so that they looked more appealing. The apps then provided users with the opportunity to share these images with others on social media. Many self-monitoring apps provided opportunities for pregnant users to enter names and photographs of themselves so that the notifications they provided can be customised. Users were thus invited to 'insert themselves' into apps so that they might better be enrolled as active users. 'Ovia Pregnancy Tracker', for instance, allowed users to add a customisable baby name and gender to the app while also adding photos and milestones.

Via the pleasures and performative qualities (rather than risk-aversion strategies) of monitoring and tracking, women were urged to 'document your special pregnancy moments and milestones' by adding photos of bellies, ultrasounds and baby showers. 'BumpDocs', as well as providing women with 'wisdom to deliver a healthy baby', also let them 'capture selfies' and share these with other pregnant women, while 'CineMama' pushed users to 'celebrate your weekly progress' by '[documenting] your pregnancy and [tracking] your belly's growth'. Taking photos of their bare stomach, women were told to turn these 'into a keepsake movie'. In conjunction with more 'serious' features such as a maternal weight tracker and following foetal growth via 'an informative video for each month of pregnancy', the app offered other features for women to 'track your memories and milestones in the app diary and personalise them with photos and our mood metre' to share in the digital world. Such features were a mainstay of many pregnancy apps on the market.

It is notable that many apps use the term baby rather than foetus, thus suggesting a stance that positions this entity as already a person. Nonetheless, foetuses themselves were often personalised in these apps. Apps like 'First Time Pregnancy', for example, contained screenshots of babies framed as 'little boxers' or as babies with their 'eyes open' who are growing larger and strengthening bones and muscles. One app, entitled 'Kick to Pick', involved placing a smartphone on a pregnant abdomen to monitor foetal kick patterns and suggesting names for the baby based on these patterns (supposedly allowing 'the whole family to get involved in the naming of your child, even the baby itself'). This configuration was enhanced via apps providing information by assuming a foetus's voice speaking from within the womb: for instance, 'Pregnancy 41 Weeks' contained information in week 9 starting with 'Hi Mom. I am growing'.

Here, we can see how apps constructed pregnancy as pleasure (or 'thrill') but also blurred the boundary between risk-avoiding practices and entertainment. Another example of this is apps which allowed women to monitor a foetal heartbeat or movement ('kicks'). The app 'Fetal Doppler UnbornHeart', with 100,000–500,000 downloads from Google Play, allowed users to 'share the joy of expecting a baby with your loved ones'. The developers of this app – used with a mini-Doppler ultrasound attachment for the smartphone sold by the same company – described it as making 'listening to your baby's heartbeat an entertaining and social experience by providing a way to record the foetal heart sounds and to share them with your family and friends [...] via e-mail, text message, Facebook and Twitter'.

Together with similar apps on the market (such as 'Cocoon Life Pregnancy', 'BabyScope', 'Flutter', 'My Baby's Beat', 'SKEEPER Fetal Heart Rate', 'BabyWatch', 'Lullabeats' and 'Tiny Beats'), monitoring and listening to foetal heart rates was configured as an 'entertaining and social experience' to share with family and friends using various digital resources. In so doing, mothers and fathers were expected to 'bond' and 'connect with her unborn baby', with a father's absence of embodied knowledge, in particular, being framed as a diminished capacity to connect with their baby. Likewise, the 'Baby HeartScope Doppler' app gave parents the opportunity to 'bond with your baby before he is born' and to 'hear your baby hiccup, swallow, move, kick, push, tap and roll'. According to the description, the app also allowed parents to predict the baby's gender and let siblings hear the heartbeat 'so that they can be happy about their new sister or brother'. In such apps, the serious (medical) and playful (social) boundaries of apps became muddied (see Lupton & Thomas, 2015, for further discussion of pregnancy games).

Discussion

In this article, we have examined an interesting and important issue: that is, the ways in which pregnancy apps frame pregnancy as a period of danger (which they can help mitigate) and as a period of pleasure (which they can help enhance). The new modes of portraying pregnancy represented by the apps we analysed here bring together the private with the public spheres, the commercial with the personal, in unprecedented ways. As we have demonstrated, a discourse of risk and responsibilisation is central to these apps. The pregnant body has increasingly become a highly public and tightly monitored condition. Risk discourse brings out social accounting practices in particularly forceful ways (Horlick-Jones, 2005); it becomes a 'forensic resource [...] a language with which to hold persons accountable' (Douglas, 1992, p. 22). In this context, women must contain risks to, and be solely responsible for, both the foetus and the pregnant body, with risk – connected with apparatuses of biopolitics in neoliberal societies creating docile and productive bodies – emerging at various levels of meaning from the structural to the cultural and symbolic (Lupton, 2012).

Pregnancy has increasingly become both a highly public and a tightly monitored condition, with women invited to take up a diverse array of discourses and practices focusing on how they deploy and manage their pregnant bodies (Burton-Jeangros, 2011; Lupton, 2012, 2013; Ruhl, 1999; Weir, 2006). Since pregnancy is both a public and a private activity and has been increasingly colonised by processes of medicalisation, women are 'policed' and become vulnerable to advice, criticism and surveillance (Burton-Jeangros, 2011; Longhurst, 2005; Nash, 2013). Pregnancy involves heavily prescriptive moral codes of expected behaviour administered through a scrutinising public gaze depicting pregnant women as fragile and as in critical need of intervention, especially to negotiate risks – before a baby is even born – viewed as calculable and preventable (Burton-Jeangros, 2011; Lupton, 2012, 2013; Warren & Brewis, 2004).

Our critical analysis of pregnancy apps has shown that many of these apps seek to fulfil a similar function. Located in a context of neoliberalism and disciplinary power valorising self-tracking and the generation and display of personal biometrics, apps can afford close and highly detailed self-monitoring of pregnant and foetal bodies and facilitate the sharing of these data with others. Our analysis suggests that perhaps now more than ever, pregnant women and the unborn have become highly visible, aestheticised and monitored, both for medical and for entertainment and consumption purposes. While apps may be used for connectivity and convenient access to a mass of information, they may also play a crucial role in the everyday practices of the contemporary maternal subject. We have already noted the popularity and common use of such apps by the current generation of pregnant women in countries such as the United States, Australia and Ireland. Apps arguably constitute one more regime of ritual purity in the avid pursuit of attaining a 'normal' and idealised pregnancy outcome. Not only may the apps arouse feelings of anxiety, self-responsibility and blame, but they also may offer a solution for women, who are entirely accountable for maternal and foetal health (Landsman, 2009; Lupton, 2013; Sutherland, 2010), as part of their sales pitch (that is, this will keep you/ your baby safe).

Equally, as we have shown, many pregnancy apps offer entertainment and construct pregnancy as a social event. Taken together, we have shown how the apps loosely categorised as 'thrills' – games and heartbeat/movement monitors particularly – are premised on notions of consumption and playfulness. Beneath these obvious notions, however, lie more problematic assumptions and normative expectations. First, they rely on heteronormative and gendered stereotypes related to pregnant women's (aestheticised and well-groomed) appearance and conduct as well as the expected presence of a male partner. Focusing on apps designed both explicitly and implicitly for young girls, the enactment of femininity, coupledom, parenthood and particularly motherhood is often clichéd and sexist.

We suggest that these apps for girls are deeply rooted in – and act to reproduce – cultural ideologies of female sexual beauty and heteronormative gender assumptions. They are both playful and located in a framework of stereotypic expectations of appearance and conduct. The pregnant woman depicted in these apps is represented as interested only in her appearance or the accomplishment of domestic duties and preparing for the birth of her baby while maintaining a glamorous appearance into the labour suite and beyond (we did not find any apps games for girls involving 'pregnant mommy' engaging in paid employment, for example). She is also frequently accompanied by her handsome, doting husband. The point here is that while the self-monitoring and pregnancy information apps directed at risk focus intently on the medicalised pregnant body, these games for girls portray an equally distorted view of pregnant embodiment as *ideally* highly fashionable and well-groomed.

Previous research into video games has demonstrated their highly gendered nature and the ways in which both female and male bodies in these games are portrayed using a restricted set of meanings and codes relating to hegemonic masculinities and femininities (Dickerman, Christensen, & Kerl-McClain, 2008; Thornham, 2008). Apps similarly depict a narrow and partial perspective of women's (pregnant) bodies as, ideally, primed and beautified. Men are also not immune from gendered and sexist stereotypes in apps; they are often caricatured as disinterested, bumbling sidekicks requiring training and encouragement to become an idealised father and partner.

In short, we suggest that such apps enact problematic discourses, especially when directed towards young girls. Such artefacts can be dismissed as harmless diversions yet early preconceptions of gender roles are reinforced and may, arguably, have enduring effects for educating young people about gender, parenthood and identity. We found that the apps we examined overwhelmingly do not account for family diversity. Whether directed at health monitoring and risk avoidance or for entertainment purposes, these apps tend to assume a pregnant woman who is partnered with a male who is the biological father of her child. Little awareness or representation is provided of single mothers, same-sex partners, those who achieved pregnancy using donor gametes or surrogate parenthood.

Furthermore, the types of pregnancy apps we have examined transform the foetus into babies for women and partners (transformed into parents) to enjoy and consume. This arguably becomes an expectation; celebrating transformations during a pregnancy (mostly online) and the growth, development and appearance of the foetus can become a tool for women to produce appropriate performances of pregnancy and 'successful' maternal femininity (Littler, 2013; Longhurst, 2000, 2005; Nash, 2013; Neiterman, 2012). Paying close attention to the developments in one's foetus, celebrating such changes and taking care to share details about it with others, thus, becomes a signal of appropriately involved and caring motherhood. Such apps enact pregnancy as a matter of consumption which distinguishes the unborn as a consumable entity and so a conscious and sentient (human) actor (Mitchell & Georges, 1997; Taylor, 2008) 'with its own rights and privileges' (Lupton, 2013: 9).

Apps that involve the aestheticisation of foetuses conform to broader moves towards rendering the unborn body a public entity that is celebrated for its preciousness and beauty (Kroløkke, 2010; Lupton, 2013). These spectatorship apps, much like the 'consumption' of ultrasound imaging (Kroløkke, 2010; Mitchell, 2001; Taylor, 2008), make pregnancies seem more 'real' in the absence of embodied knowledge and allow parents to rework pregnancy experiences by providing a way of knowing and feeling *their* baby. Furthermore, they frame the foetus as a separate and conscious agent; the foetus is humanised and personalised, represented as an already social, autonomous actor.

Conclusion

In this article, we have shown how apps, far from being neutral technologies which purport to simply providing information and advice (as well as entertaining opportunities), represent women's bodies in problematic ways. The two distinct forms of pregnancy apps that we identified (those based around 'threats' and those around 'thrills') are not necessarily mutually exclusive. Taken together, the apps rest on neoliberal ideologies concerning the management and responsibilisation of the self/body. Whether they are explicitly directed at the identification and containment of pregnancy-related risk or at ludifying pregnancy, users of the apps are encouraged to view pregnancy as an embodied mode of close monitoring and surveillance, display and performance. Our analysis has also highlighted how pregnancy increasingly becomes a marketable moment. This is not an entirely new development, but it has been assumed swiftly by apps. A key example here is apps which allow parents to monitor foetal movement and heartbeats. In conjunction with other apps framing pregnancy as a risky condition requiring intervention, foetal heartbeat/kick monitors offer a solution, commonly supplemented by the purchase of a 'personal' foetal Doppler available on online shopping sites.

In the past, pregnant women have been offered many forms of media as part of encouraging them to learn about and perform pregnancy. We suggest that what makes apps different, and more potent, are the following: their sheer volume (with more apps released onto the market regularly); their accessibility both in relation to economics (often available to download free-of-charge) and their convenience (anyone with a mobile device, such as a smartphone or tablet, can download apps and use them across temporal and spatial locations); the near-absent regulation of app developers and the content that they create and their huge implications for data security and privacy.

As is the case with other medical and health apps, the monitoring and regulation of pregnancy apps, given their proliferation, remains a challenge for regulatory bodies (Yetisen et al., 2014). The UK Government has released guidance on apps and other standalone medical devices under the policy of 'patient safety' (MHRA 2014). Exploring and evaluating whether this government guidance and associated regulatory frameworks are well-equipped enough to handle the wealth of apps currently on the market, not just for pregnancy but for health more broadly, is of paramount importance. So too, the implications for users of data security and privacy issues deserve further attention. Several studies have revealed the ways in which the often very private information that people upload to apps (regularly simply as part of agreeing to terms and conditions when downloading apps) is subject to data breaches and exploitation by app developers and third parties to whom they sell these data (Ackerman, 2013; Huckvale, Prieto, Tilney, Benghozi, & Car, 2015). These problems are also evident with pregnancy apps (Dembosky, 2013; Scott, Gome, Richards, & Caldwell, 2015).

As for the relationship between pregnancy and apps as a new form of digital media, much ground remains uncovered. Though many apps are on the market little scholarly focus has been directed towards these digital media artefacts, this is a crucial and timely opportunity to examine the interactions between expectant parents and these technologies, particularly with respect to how they use them, what impact they have on their experiences of pregnancy and how they draw on, reproduce and initiate new discourses of performing parenthood. This, we argue, will reveal vital insights for uncovering the relationship between health, risk, society and digital technologies.

Disclosure statement

No potential conflict of interest was reported by the authors.

Funding

Gareth Thomas would like to thank Deborah Lupton and the University of Canberra for funding a visiting fellowship supporting the conduct of the research reported in this article.

References

Ackerman, L. (2013). *Mobile health and fitness applications and information privacy*. San Diego, CA: Privacy Rights Clearing House.

Burton-Jeangros, C. (2011). Surveillance of risks in everyday life: The agency of pregnant women and its limitations. *Social Theory & Health, 9*(4), 419–436. doi:10.1057/sth.2011.15

Coxon, K. (2014). Risk in pregnancy and birth: Are we talking to ourselves? *Health, Risk & Society, 16*(6), 481–493. doi:10.1080/13698575.2014.957262

Declercq, E., Sakala, C., Corry, M., Applebaum, S., & Herrlich, A. (2013). *Listening to mothers III: Pregnancy and birth*. New York: Childbirth Connection.

Dembosky, A. (2013, July 17 2014). Pregnancy apps raise fresh privacy concerns. *The Financial Times*. Retrieved from http://www.ft.com/cms/s/0/1c560432-2782-11e3-ae16-00144feab7de.html#axzz37gHqmHO7

Derbyshire, E., & Dancey, D. (2013). Smartphone medical applications for women's health: What is the evidence-base and feedback? *International Journal of Telemedicine and Applications, 2013*. doi:10.1155/2013/782074

Dickerman, C., Christensen, J., & Kerl-McClain, S. B. (2008). Big breasts and bad guys: Depictions of gender and race in video games. *Journal of Creativity in Mental Health, 3*(1), 20–29. doi:10.1080/15401380801995076

Doty, J. L., & Dworkin, J. (2014). Online social support for parents: A critical review. *Marriage & Family Review, 50*(2), 174–198. doi:10.1080/01494929.2013.834027

Douglas, M. (1992). *Risk and blame: Essays in cultural theory*. London: Routledge.

Fairclough, N., Mulderrig, J., & Wodak, R. (2011). Critical discourse analysis. In T. van Dijk (Ed.), *Discourse studies: A multidisciplinary introduction* (pp. 357–378). London, UK: Sage.

Frissen, V., Lammes, S., De Lange, M., De Mul, J., & Raessens, J. (Eds). (2015). *Playful identities: The ludification of digital media cultures*. Amsterdam: Amsterdam University Press.

Hearn, L., Miller, M., & Fletcher, A. (2013). Online healthy lifestyle support in the perinatal period: What do women want and do they use it? *Australian Journal of Primary Health, 19* (4), 313–318. doi:10.1071/PY13039

Hearn, L., Miller, M., & Lester, L. (2014). Reaching perinatal women online: The healthy you, healthy baby website and app. *Journal of Obesity*. doi:10.1155/2014/573928

Horlick-Jones, T. (2005). On 'risk work': Professional discourse, accountability, and everyday action. *Health, Risk & Society, 7*(3), 293–307. doi:10.1080/13698570500229820

Huckvale, K., Prieto, J., Tilney, M., Benghozi, P.-J., & Car, J. (2015). Unaddressed privacy risks in accredited health and wellness apps: A cross-sectional systematic assessment. *BMC Medicine, 13*(1). Retrieved September 6, 2015, from http://www.biomedcentral.com/1741-7015/13/214

Jahns, R.-G. (2014, September 16) The 8 drivers and barriers that will shape the mHealth app market in the next 5 years. *research2guidance*. Retrieved from http://mhealtheconomics.com/the-8-drivers-and-barriers-that-will-shape-the-mhealth-app-market-in-the-next-5-years/

Johnson, S. (2014). "Maternal devices", social media and the self-management of pregnancy, mothering and child health. *Societies, 4*(2), 330–350. doi:10.3390/soc4020330

Kraschnewski, L. J., Chuang, H. C., Poole, S. E., Peyton, T., Blubaugh, I., Pauli, J., & Reddy, M. (2014). Paging "Dr. Google": Does technology fill the gap created by the prenatal care visit structure? Qualitative focus group study with pregnant women. *Journal of Medical Internet Research, 16*(6), e147. Retrieved from http://www.jmir.org/2014/6/e147/

Kroløkke, C. (2010). On a trip to the womb: Biotourist metaphors in fetal ultrasound imaging. *Women's Studies in Communication, 33*(2), 138–153. doi:10.1080/07491409.2010.507577

Landsman, G. (2009). *Reconstructing motherhood and disability in the age of 'perfect' babies: Lives of mothers and infants and toddlers with disabilities*. New York: Routledge.

Littler, J. (2013). The rise of the 'yummy mummy': Popular conservatism and the neoliberal maternal in contemporary British culture. *Communication, Culture & Critique, 6*(2), 227–243. doi:10.1111/cccr.2013.6.issue-2

Longhurst, R. (2000). Corporeographies' of pregnancy: 'bikini babes. *Environment and Planning D: Society and Space, 18*(4), 453–472. doi:10.1068/d234

Longhurst, R. (2005). *Maternities: Gender, bodies and space.* London: Routledge.

Lupton, D. (2012). 'Precious cargo': Foetal subjects, risk and reproductive citizenship. *Critical Public Health, 22*(3), 329–340. doi:10.1080/09581596.2012.657612

Lupton, D. (2013). *The social worlds of the unborn.* Houndmills: Palgrave Macmillan.

Lupton, D. (2014a). Critical perspectives on digital health technologies. *Sociology Compass, 8*(12), 1344–1359. doi:10.1111/soc4.12226

Lupton, D. (2014b). Apps as artefacts: Towards a critical perspective on mobile health and medical apps. *Societies, 4*(4), 606–622. doi:10.3390/soc4040606

Lupton, D. (2015a). Health promotion in the digital era: A critical commentary. *Health Promotion International, 30*(1), 174–183. doi:10.1093/heapro/dau091

Lupton, D. (2015b). Quantified sex: A critical analysis of sexual and reproductive self-tracking using apps. *Culture, Health & Sexuality, 17*(4), 440–453. doi:10.1080/13691058.2014.920528

Lupton, D., & Jutel, A. (2015). 'It's like having a physician in your pocket!' A critical analysis of self-diagnosis smartphone apps. *Social Science & Medicine, 133*, 128–135. doi:10.1016/j.socscimed.2015.04.004

Lupton, D., & Thomas, G. M. (2015). Playing pregnancy: The ludification and gamification of expectant motherhood in smartphone apps. *M/C Journal, 18*(5). Retrieved from http://journal.media-culture.org.au/index.php/mcjournal/article/viewArticle/1012

Medicines and Healthcare Products Regulatory Agency (MHRA). (2014). *Medical device stand-alone software including apps.* London: The Stationery Office (TSO).

Mitchell, L. (2001). *Baby's first picture: Ultrasound and the politics of fetal subjects.* Toronto: University of Toronto Press.

Mitchell, L. M., & Georges, E. (1997). Cross-cultural cyborgs: Greek and Canadian women's discourses on fetal ultrasound. *Feminist Studies, 23*(2), 373–401. doi:10.2307/3178405

Nash, M. (2013). *Making 'postmodern' mothers: Pregnant embodiment, baby bumps and body image.* Houndmills: Palgrave Macmillan.

Neiterman, E. (2012). Doing pregnancy: Pregnant embodiment as performance. *Women's Studies International Forum, 35*(5), 372–383. doi:10.1016/j.wsif.2012.07.004

O'Higgins, A., Murphy, O. C., Egan, A., Mullaney, L., Sheehan, S., & Turner, M. J. (2014). The use of digital media by women using the maternity services in a developed country. *Irish Medical Journal, 107*(10), 313–315.

Peyton, T., Poole, E., Reddy, M., Kraschnewski, J., & Chuang, C. (2014). *Every pregnancy is different: Designing mHealth for the pregnancy ecology.* Proceedings of the 2014 conference on Designing Interactive Systems, ACM, 577–586.

Rich, E., & Miah, A. (2014). Understanding digital health as public pedagogy: A critical framework. *Societies, 4*(2), 296–315. Retrieved from http://www.mdpi.com/2075-4698/4/2/296

Robinson, F., & Jones, C. (2014). Women's engagement with mobile device applications in pregnancy and childbirth. *The Practising Midwife, 17*(1), 23–25.

Rodger, D., Skuse, A., Wilmore, M., Humphreys, S., Dalton, J., Flabouris, M., & Clifton, V. L. (2013). Pregnant women's use of information and communications technologies to access pregnancy-related health information in South Australia. *Australian Journal of Primary Health, 19*(4), 308–312. doi:10.1071/PY13029

Ruhl, L. (1999). Liberal governance and prenatal care: Risk and regulation in pregnancy. *Economy and Society, 28*(1), 95–117. doi:10.1080/03085149900000026

Scott, K., Gome, G., Richards, D., & Caldwell, P. H. Y. (2015). How trustworthy are apps for maternal and child health? *Health and Technology, 4*(4), 329–336. doi:10.1007/s12553-015-0099-x

Seneviratne, S., Seneviratne, A., Mohapatra, P., & Mahanti, A. (2015). Your installed apps reveal your gender and more! *Mobile Computing and Communications Review, 18*(3), 55–61. doi:10.1145/2721896

Statista. (2015a, June 26). Cumulative number of apps downloaded from the Apple App Store from July 2008 to June 2015 (in billions). *Statista Inc.* Retrieved from http://www.statista.com/statistics/263794/number-of-downloads-from-the-apple-app-store/

Statista. (2015b, June 26). Number of apps available in leading app stores as of May 2015. *Statista Inc*. Retrieved from http://www.statista.com/statistics/276623/number-of-apps-available-in-leading-app-stores/.

Sutherland, J.-A. (2010). Mothering, guilt and shame. *Sociology Compass, 4*, 310–321. doi:10.1111/(ISSN)1751-9020

Taylor, J. (2008). *The public life of the fetal sonogram: Technology, consumption and the politics of reproduction*. New Brunswick, NJ: Rutgers University Press.

Thornham, H. (2008). It's a boy thing. *Feminist Media Studies, 8*(2), 127–142. doi:10.1080/14680770801980505

Tripp, N., Hainey, K., Liu, A., Poulton, A., Peek, M., Kim, J., & Nanan, R. (2014). An emerging model of maternity care: Smartphone, midwife, doctor? *Women and Birth, 27*(1), 64–67. doi:10.1016/j.wombi.2013.11.001

Warren, S., & Brewis, J. (2004). Matter over mind? Examining the experience of pregnancy. *Sociology, 38*(2), 219–236. doi:10.1177/0038038504040860

Weir, L. (2006). *Pregnancy, risk, and biopolitics: On the threshold of the living subject*. London: Routledge.

Yetisen, A. K., Martinez-Hurtado, J., da Cruz Vasconcellos, F., Simsekler, M. C. E., Akram, M. S., & Lowe, C. R. (2014). The regulation of mobile medical applications. *Lab on a Chip, 14*(5), 833–840. doi:10.1039/c3lc51235e

Asthma on the move: how mobile apps remediate risk for disease management

Alison Kenner

Department of Politics, Drexel University, Philadelphia, USA

Mobile health apps have emerged as a technological fix promising to improve asthma management. In the United States, treatment non-adherence has become the most pressing asthma risk; as such, emphasis has increasingly focused on getting asthmatics to take medications as prescribed. In this article I examine how mobile Asthma (mAsthma) apps operate as part of digital risk society, where mobile apps create new modes of risk identification and management; promise to control messy and undisciplined subjects and care practices; use algorithms to generate new risk calculations; and make risk livelier through digital assemblages. Drawing on ethnographic fieldwork, content analysis of mAsthma app design, as well as interviews with app developers, in this article I argue that these digital care technologies strip disease and risk of biographical, ecological and affective detail in ways that largely reinforce biomedical paradigms. Yet some apps offer new insight into the place-based dynamics of environmental health, a view made possible with digitised personal tracking, visual analytics and crowdsourced data. mAsthma apps are caught in the tension between the biopolitics of existing chronic care infrastructure, which reinforce a strict neoliberalised patient responsibility, and the promise of collective, place-based approaches to global environmental health problems.

Introduction

Chronic disease management is often anchored by self-monitoring practices and daily pharmaceutical regimes. Biomedical guidelines for asthma management fit this formula, but there are key differences between asthma and other chronic disease conditions: Asthma symptoms are triggered by environmental exposures tied to place-based contexts. Many asthmatics manage their disease using both environmental control practices and medications that mitigate symptoms pre-emptively or at the moment of exposure. In biomedical and public health paradigms, however, ad hoc management strategies are seen as risky; adherence to daily controller medication is viewed as the most effective means of reducing or preventing symptoms. Thus, in US asthma care arenas, non-adherence to treatment is seen as the most pressing asthma risk; as such, emphasis has increasingly focused on getting asthmatics to take medications as prescribed.

In step with the rapid growth of the smartphone market, mobile health apps have emerged as a technological fix promising to improve asthma management. Although a broad and diverse market, mobile asthma (mAsthma) apps promise to address key challenges related to non-adherence. Many apps aim to bolster health literacy, enabling users to better identify environmental and behavioural risks that trigger symptoms; routinise disease management and increase use of controller medicines; and make patient–provider communication more efficient. In this way, mAsthma apps build on, extend and refine existing disease management regimes through personal technologies that remediate asthma risk in 'particular techno-semiotic networks' (van Loon, 2014, p. 444); this is achieved as digital platforms draw together disease management guidelines and personal health data in real-time analytics that point users towards some risks and not others (Bolter & Grusin, 1999; Lupton, 2016). The apps do more than communicate asthma risks; they make them performative, immediate and networked.

In this article, I examine how mAsthma apps operate as part of digital risk society, where mobile apps create new modes of risk identification and management; promise to control messy and undisciplined subjects and care practices; use algorithms to generate new risk calculations; and make risk livelier through digital assemblages (Lupton, 2016). Drawing on ethnographic fieldwork, content analysis of mAsthma app design, as well as interviews with app developers, in this article I argue that these digital care technologies strip disease and risk of biographical, ecological and affective detail in ways that largely reinforce biomedical paradigms. Yet some apps offer new insight into the place-based dynamics of environmental health, a view made possible with digitised personal tracking, visual analytics and crowdsourced data. mAsthma apps are caught in the tension between the biopolitics of existing chronic care infrastructure (Langstrup, 2013), which reinforce a strict neoliberalised patient responsibility, and the promise of collective, place-based approaches to global environmental health problems.

Asthma, risk and digital health studies

Asthma, risk and emplaced care

Asthma is an environmental health condition with global prevalence rates exceeding 300 million people worldwide (The Global Asthma Network, 2014). A heterogeneous, variable, yet chronic disease condition, asthma is characterised by disordered breathing that includes wheezing, coughing, chest tightness and shortness of breath. The intensity of symptoms can range from a distracting nuisance to events that disrupt daily activities, and in its most severe form, accelerate into life-threatening events. Asthma symptoms can be triggered by common domestic objects, local environmental conditions and even a handful of activities. Dust mites, tobacco smoke, pollen, pests, outdoor air pollution, cleaning products, cold air, exercise and stress are commonly cited triggers. Such exposures are understood as asthma risks with potential to produce symptoms and full-blown attacks. In this article, I define asthma risk as objects, contexts and behaviours that have the potential to produce asthma symptoms and attacks. This definition is different from the biomedical definition of risk factors, which include a broader range of factors such as genetic and hereditary dynamics associated with an individual's susceptibility to asthma. There is no cure for asthma; those who suffer from the condition manage symptoms using a variety of biomedical and environmental control practices that I refer to as *emplaced care*.

Reno described emplacement as 'the material, experiential, and discursive process through which places are creatively elaborated' (2011, p. 517). Emplacement describes embodied and affective boundary-making practices that community members and patients use to identify things out of place, such as environmental hazards that leak or seep into public and domestic spaces in ways that produce health risks. Emplacement has also been used to illustrate how medication and medical products become embedded in care settings (Hodgetts, Chamberlain, Gabe, & Dew, 2011; Langstrup, 2013; Lehoux, Saint-Arnaud, & Richard, 2004). The way care technologies (including medication) are emplaced in homes, clinics and on mobile bodies both derives from and shapes how disease is understood, experienced and managed. Emplacement practices – whether in the context of sensing and identifying environmental hazards, or experiencing and managing disease – are often conditioned by perceptions of risk.

Asthmatics practise emplaced care when their responses to disease stem from the environmental and temporal dynamics of their illness. Emplaced care is anchored by 'body-ecologies' in place, a term that describes the materially porous and intermingled relationship between human biology and environments (Murphy, 2006). In interviews, many asthmatics describe how they use embodied and affective knowledge to detect environmental triggers (Kenner, 2013); their bodies act as sensors that alert them to risky body–ecology relations (Murphy, 2006; Shapiro, 2015). Environmental control practices – such as leaving a place that poses a risk to health, cleaning the home routinely, avoiding locations or objects that produce symptoms, and purchasing products that mitigate triggers (such as air filters, dust covers and organic cleaning products) – are forms of emplaced care derived from affective knowledge that links disease to environmental risk. Asthmatics sense and interact with environments to produce understanding of risk, and by extension, care responses; this includes the temporal dimensions of disease, such as past symptom experiences and memories, present sensations and interactions, as well as possible futures (Lupton, 2013c; Stewart, 2011). In some contexts, however, disordered breathing emerges too quickly and forcefully for environmental control practices to sufficiently mitigate symptoms. In such situations, asthmatics must use a rescue inhaler with medication that opens airways to relieve symptoms.

Given that atmospheric composition of indoor and outdoor places is constantly changing – daily, with seasonal change, and even year to year – environmental control practices are not enough to prevent asthma symptoms and exacerbations. Living in constant risk of disordered breathing is miserable, disruptive and sometimes life threatening. Although awareness of environmental conditions can aid disease management, it is difficult, if not impossible, to always know the qualities of place and what an individual might be exposed to. Environmental uncertainty, and by extension, health risks, can be managed with daily controller medications that reduce airway inflammation and make the body less responsive to environmental exposures. Many asthmatics are prescribed daily controller medications as a primary risk reduction strategy; environmental control practices are meant to supplement pharmaceutical regimes as a secondary risk management strategy (NACI, 2013). In biomedical and public health paradigms, daily medication use is the optimal response to uncertainty, heterogeneity and dynamic body-ecologies; the most effective means of controlling asthma risk.

Like many chronic disease conditions, however, adherence to treatment regimes, such as taking medication routinely as prescribed and monitoring pulmonary performance, is relatively low among asthmatics. The variable nature of asthma lends itself to non-adherence; the absence of symptoms leads some patients to conclude that their disease is dormant, and daily medication is no longer needed (Bender & Bender, 2005, Chambre & Goldner, 2008). Some asthmatics resist biomedical mandates by questioning the long-term effects of inhaled corticosteroid use (Bender & Bender, 2005; Chambre & Goldner, 2008). Sometimes non-adherence stems, in part, from lack of understanding about the disease condition and how medications work (Bender & Bender, 2005; Boulet, 1998).

Horne and Weinman (2002) attribute the problem of non-adherence to a disconnect between the values and knowledge of medical practitioners, and that of patients; this parallels the work of risk studies scholars who have shown that public health practitioners need to better understand the beliefs and values that underpin everyday decision-making so that health mandates can meet target audiences appropriately (Alaszewski, 2013; Foster & Heyman, 2013; Thing & Ottesen, 2013).

Non-adherence is cited as the number one reason for poor asthma outcomes, including missed work and school days, lesser quality of life, use of emergency services and death (Rand et al., 2012; Williams et al., 2004). This adds up to the economic burden of poor asthma control – if asthmatics take a controller medication daily, they will have fewer exacerbations and symptoms; they will miss work and school less, and reduce use of healthcare services such as emergency departments. Well-controlled asthma will save the healthcare system money. As an example of how seriously institutions representing experts in asthma take asthmatic non-adherence, the US National Heart, Lung, and Blood Institute's latest asthma programme, the National Asthma Control Initiative, urges clinicians, patients, caregivers, schools, employers, as well as insurers, states and non-profits to help implement six key care guidelines: use inhaled corticosteroids to control asthma; use written asthma action plans to guide patient self-management; assess asthma severity at the initial visit to determine initial treatment; assess and monitor asthma control and adjust treatment if needed; schedule follow-up visits at periodic intervals; and control environmental exposures that worsen the patient's asthma. Individual measures to limit environmental exposures to triggers barely feature in federal guidelines for controlling asthma. In the United States, the dominant response and main way of controlling asthma is pharmaceutical (Langstrup, 2013; Mitman, 2007; Whitmarsh, 2008).

However, there is low adherence to pharmaceutical regimes. Chronic disease apps are one response to this perceived problem. Most of the mAsthma apps reviewed in this article are designed to reduce risk by reinforcing treatment adherence. Yet because asthma is an environmental health condition triggered by place-based atmospheric qualities, some apps emphasise the potential of locative technology for disease management. The soft biopolitics backing the incorporations of GPS data, however, varies from one app to the next, as will be discussed (Cheney-Lippold, 2011). No matter their versatility, breadth or intricacy, all mAsthma apps use existing biomedical and public health paradigms as the basis for their assessment of asthma risk.

Risk in critical digital health studies

In an overburdened healthcare system, where business as usual fails to get patients to comply with disease management regimens, digital health technology seems to offer solutions that would improve care and cut costs (Rich & Miah, 2014). Critical digital health studies scholars, however, have shown that emerging technologies do much more than address healthcare challenges such as outcomes, expenditures, literacy and adherence; digital health platforms have disciplinary affects that reinforce dominant medical discourses, individualise responsibility for public health through self-management and consumption practices, and reconceptualise the body and relationships to corporeality (see the themed issue of *Societies*, Cakici & Sanches, 2014; Johnson, 2014; Lupton, 2014b; Rich & Miah, 2014; Ruckenstein, 2014; Sosnowy, 2014; and Till, 2014). Mobile health apps in particular focus on lifestyle factors that frame health in terms of commodity culture rather than sociocultural dimensions that produce disease, often unevenly (Rich & Miah, 2014).

Writing on the contours of digital risk society, Lupton highlights four components of risk digitisation that are particularly relevant to mAsthma apps: the development of algorithms that perform risk calculations; the identification and management of risks; a promise to exert 'control over messy, undisciplined scenarios' and subjects; and the creation of assemblages that make risk livelier – lively in the sense that risk and its perceptions are assembled through information flows and networks with a new degree of immediacy (Lupton, 2016, p. 4). Mobile apps allow users who enter and track personal health data to identify patterns of behaviour, affect and exposure that may otherwise go unnoticed; apps provide a structure that enables users to think about activities, places and outcomes in new ways. As such, these apps remediate risk: As personal technologies they demand a repetitive, sustained action from users, whose data are structured by risks remediated through app design (van Loon, 2014). Risk made digital is remediated as it is imbued with active force; remediated because it 'operates within a network that is denser – consisting of more matter-energy-information flows – than a risk whose probability exclusively travels by means of narration and therefore remains hypothetical' (van Loon, 2014, p. 450). This is particularly true of digital risk assemblages where many bits of data are reassembled by predictive algorithms – meditated from previous social, political and cultural frames of risk (Cheney-Lippold, 2011). More than narrations on the page, risk made digital draws mobile app users into the process of making risks real, and personal, through self-tracking and locative technologies; digital affect is produced through the accumulation of personal data over time and place. Embedded in digital society, health apps make risk lively and vital through multiplication, circulation and intersection with other actors and datum across networks whose political import must be considered (Lupton, 2016).

Many health apps draw users' embodied knowledge and experience into digital remediation. These apps condition users 'to use information *about* their bodies in accordance with the affective responses to that information' (Rich & Miah, 2014, p. 309). Data visualisations become an important means through which to engage the body and reshape behaviour. In these apps, the body is disassembled and channelled into databases and data flows, then reassembled in visual analytics that categorise the user in ways that often call for intervention (Haggerty & Ericson, 2000; Ruckenstein, 2014). These 'data doubles' prompt users to respond to numbers made visual, which stand for health or disease, 'decorporealized and decontextualized bodies – hybrid composites of information – in ways that are intended to encourage people to act in certain ways' (Ruckenstein, 2014, p. 71). Data doubles, of course, are lively and dynamic, even if cast within biopolitical logics that push neoliberal care practices. In mHealth apps specifically, affective learning works for neoliberal agendas; information, design and affect prompt users to control body and behaviour in line with dominant cultural values (Johnson, 2014; Lupton, 2013a, 2014a; Rich & Miah, 2014; Ruckenstein, 2014).

The self-surveillance practices that these mobile health apps enable are designed to work at the level of subject formation, where disease data entered by individuals is compared and visualised against biomedical benchmarks that dictate normal, healthy metrics (French & Smith, 2013; Holt, 2013). mHealth converts surveillance systems into neoliberal products where users can consume and help produce a biopolitical health culture (Lupton, 2013a, 2013b). Personal tracking moves risk calculations that govern uncertainty to handheld surveillance platforms where users are trained to think and act on future health risks based on biomedical algorithms (Cheney-Lippold, 2011;

Dumit, 2012). Quantified lifestyles and behaviours get cast numerically, in visual form, in ways that carry more weight than social determinants of health (Cakici & Sanches, 2014; Lupton, 2013b). In the case of asthma, an environmental health problem produced in part by poor housing stock, chemicals, air pollution and climate change (Brown et al., 2003; Fortun et al., 2014; Gold & Wright, 2005), mAsthma apps distribute public, environmental risks to the social body through patients who are told to take personal responsibility for their disease (French & Smith, 2013). Design choices that privilege risky behaviours and lifestyle factors, often render invisible 'local and context-dependent knowledge' (Cakici & Sanches, 2014, p. 400) that would otherwise implicate a failed governance of the commons (Carlsson & Sandström, 2008). Yet alongside analyses that point to the biopolitical and neoliberal affects of these emerging technologies, critical digital health studies scholars also highlight social practices – the creation of virtual communities, enhanced modes of awareness and access to information and services – that could provide openings for new modes of collective care (Martin, Myers, & Viseu, 2015).

Considering the number of mAsthma apps on the market, there is little data on how widely asthma management apps are used among asthmatics – a strange data gap considering these personal health technologies are marketed as information rich tools that can improve health outcomes for patients, caregivers, doctors and public health agencies. Nevertheless, analysis of the design and development of mAsthma apps – which is the focus of this article – lends insight into how emerging health technology fits within existing chronic care infrastructures (Langstrup, 2013). In this article, I analyse the design of mAsthma app platforms, asking how the structure, function and communication pathways of these personal health technologies reinforce or depart from dominant biomedical logics and practices.

Methodology

In this article I draw on data from an ethnographic study of asthma care in the United States. My analysis of the mAsthma market began in 2010 when several apps appeared in health technology news, most notably *Asthmapolis* (Marsan, 2010). In December 2014, I initiated a structured investigation of the mAsthma app market. This began with a search for 'asthma' in Apple's App Store as well as Google Play; this search returned nearly 300 results from 17 countries. Between January and April 2015, I reviewed 275 apps in a preliminary content analysis (211 from Apple's App Store and 64 from Google Play); only apps available in English were reviewed. I collected data on the app release (Apple) or update date (Google), the type of seller (software developer, health clinic, university researcher or medical technology company, for example), the geographic location of the seller, the cost of the app, the number of ratings or reviews, the in-store category, the description of the app, and in the case of Google Play, the number of installations. Based on this data and content analysis of in-store descriptions, screenshots and supporting websites, I placed each app in one of seven analytic categories: compliant care, environmental care, environmental health, health literacy, integrative medicine, medical education and participatory epidemiology. I categorised mAsthma app according to four criteria: the aim of the app – to provide health information or to serve as a disease diary, for example; whether the app allowed the user to enter illness and disease management data, and if the data could be shared with the care team; whether the app used locational services and/or pulled in local environmental information; and if user data are crowdsourced and included as part of a data set intended to show asthma prevalence and incidence across a geographic area. Given the number of search results, categorisation became an important means to focus further study and analysis.

I selected 24 apps from the final three categories – compliant care, environmental health and participatory epidemiology – for more substantive content analysis on an iPhone or Android device. Three of the 24 apps required access codes that prevented further analysis; an access code requirement meant that the app was either in a testing phase and not yet publicly available, or was part of a clinical study. I also conducted in-depth interviews with software developers, doctors or marketing staff from organisations developing mAsthma apps. In addition to the initial classification criteria, design analysis attended to how apps reproduced and modified existing asthma care regimes. I paid particular attention to how each app measured and communicated risk, as well as how the app emphasised different care practices (medication use versus environmental control).

- *Compliant care apps*, in essence, function as a digital disease diary where asthmatic users can log symptoms, pulmonary performance and medication use. Some provide relatively few fields for user input: the date, peak flow reading, the previous day's dose of controller medication, use of a quick relief inhaler, symptom severity and triggers, for example. These data may be visually represented as colour-coded analytics that enable users to see disease and care at a glance, but remediated through databases and analytics that position triggers, symptoms and medication in relation to each other over time, and measured against biomedical benchmarks. Some apps also provide fields for the user to add notes to supplement quantitative inputs. Some apps enable users to add automated notifications as reminders to take medication and report pulmonary performance.
- *Environmental health apps* have all the features of advanced compliant care apps – users record symptoms, medication use, triggers and observations of daily living – but also leverage location information, either through a manually entered zip or postal code or by enabling GPS. Locative information allows the app to layer environmental, place-based and user health data. Assembling data in this way makes relationships between place and user visible. Two apps fell into the category of participatory epidemiology, a term that Freifeld et al. (2010) used to describe emerging technologies that crowdsource personal data for public health agendas.
- *Participatory epidemiology apps* geocode user data, for those who anonymously opt-in, and send data to third-party analysts. Participatory epidemiology apps are environmental health apps that share the locative data for user symptoms, triggers and medication. As the category name suggests, these apps begin to move care beyond the individual user for broad-based public health application; they work to characterise communities and places, not just the individual user experiences.

Although Google Play shows the number of downloads for each app (Apple's App Store does not), this number says nothing about how and the extent to which apps are adopted. Of the developers interviewed, all indicated that their mAsthma projects were not positioned to evaluate use, yet. Number and location of downloads, as well as anecdotal emails, were the extent of data accessible to developers. Two exceptions to this data absence occurred when a patient brought the app into clinical appointments to discuss with a provider on the development team, and when use data were collected during pre-market development, in small-scale studies. My interviews and analysis of product websites indicated that development teams are moving to build use analytics into project management, but privacy continues to be a huge barrier. Thus, the following section focuses analysis on the content and design of a compliant care app; the frameworks and actions through which risk is remediated. The following section complements this analysis with perspectives from mAsthma development team members.

Findings

The target user of mAsthma apps is the asthmatic patient, both adults and children. Some apps are geared towards the patient plus their healthcare provider or a team of caregivers responsible for a child with asthma. Participatory epidemiology apps were geared towards broader public health goals where researchers, local policymakers and epidemiologists were part of the user group. At least one app was designed for insurance companies specifically. Most mAsthma apps are free or have a free version. Paid versions offered ad free use of the app and in some cases additional features. A total of 39 apps required a fee of $10.00 or less (12 apps from the Google Play store and 27 from the iTunes Store). A handful of mAsthma apps have been developed in the university context or in collaboration with academic researchers. The vast majority of apps, however, were developed by commercial organisations: mobile app developers, medical technology companies or physician groups, for example. In some cases, apps were developed through partnerships between these groups.

When compared to other forms of digital health technologies, including apps paired with wearable devices, the cost of mAsthma is much less prohibitive. Rather than advancing new modes of treatment, mAsthma apps are positioned to bolster existing clinical practices, such as routinising medication use and doctor visits, tracking pulmonary performance, or improving patient literacy. In the clinic, information exported from the app and shared with doctors provides a record that reduces the need to rely on patient memory in clinical assessment. A number of apps were designed to collect data on the asthmatic population, an illness group that has historically frustrated the medical gaze given the variable, inconsistent and ephemeral nature of the disease (Lancet, 2008; Whitmarsh, 2008). Only one mAsthma app hinged on use of a wearable, in this case a GPS tracking device appended to the user's rescue inhaler; the wearable automatically recorded the time and location of quick-relief inhaler use and then transmitted geospatial data in real time to a remote server.

Most mAsthma apps are promoted as disease education and/or management tools; their functionality as such is premised on the risk of low health literacy and non-adherence, which are needed for well-controlled asthma. Almost all compliant care apps utilise asthma action plans, a biomedical disease management tool that provides numbers-based instruction for pharmaceutical and self-monitoring regimes. Asthma action plans emerged at the height of 1990s media coverage and awareness campaigns focused on the US epidemic. These documents are designed to help patients visualise when their disease is poorly managed and to provide instructions on course correcting, such as taking more medication within a specified time frame, increasing the frequency of peak flow readings, and seeking medical help in an urgent care or emergency unit. Typically a single-sided page, the plan categorises levels of asthma control into three colour-coded sections: green for well-controlled, yellow as a warning and red to indicate the threat of poor asthma control. Some plans even utilise the iconic traffic signal to help bolster categorical meaning. The documents in and of themselves are designed to raise 'red flags' for patients and their caregivers in everyday life (Cott & Tierney, 2013). They are exemplars of biomedical risk communication, and most mAsthma apps are modelled from these risk management treatment plans, including App J, which will be used to describe and analyse fundamental mAsthma app features.

Asthma care made digital

App J developers used the Global Initiative for Asthma control template for their app control assessment. Global Initiative for Asthma is an international organisation that was established following the US asthma epidemic in 1993. Its parent organisations are the US National Heart, Lung and Blood Institute, the US National Institutes of Health and the World Health Organization. Its work focuses on public health communication. *App J* begins as many compliant care apps do: by asking the user what kind of medication they treat their asthma with. The user enters the name and category of medication – 'regular' for maintenance inhalers or as needed for a rescue inhaler – followed by the frequency of intake and dosage. It also allows users to add notifications that remind one to take their daily controller medication. After entering prescription information, a screen pops up with an 'Important Note' – the user should only enter in dosage and frequency as prescribed by a doctor, a pharmacist or the drug manufacturer. An obligatory product message that works to remind users that everyone must follow the rules of medicine, rules that must be set and dictated by medical experts. App users enter information from their prescribed asthma action plan, but the disclaimer conveys that the user must enter this information correctly, and follow it. The app is not a doctor, and neither are developers, one interlocutor told me.

Once medications have been entered into *App J*, the user can navigate to 'Options' where they can enter in reminders – such as to take medication, to refill prescriptions, to visit the doctor and to 'check' their disease. Notification features are present in many mAsthma apps; it is part of what makes mobile apps appealing and valuable. In an interview with Jay, a medical provider who helped develop one of the mAsthma apps reviewed, smartphones were described as a personal technology that had affective value 'I wish they would take their medication like they take their phones around.' Smartphones are always with the user, and could be used to strengthen treatment practices. Those developing the app anticipate that if medication reminders are pushed through the phone, for example, adherence will improve. They use this functionality to directly address the erratic form of non-adherence, when patients forget to take their medication; it also prompts asthmatics who are rationally non-adherent to rethink their choices about modifying medication use (van Boven, Trappenburg, van der Molen, & Chavannes, 2015).

The defining feature of *App J*, however, is the 'Check', which takes users through a five-question asthma control assessment. The first question asks the user if, in the past week, they have had asthma symptoms more than twice during the day; the user simply answers by selecting 'yes' or 'no'. The second question asks if the user has needed rescue medication more than twice in the last week; again, users answer with a 'yes' or 'no' response. The same structure is used for the final three questions: limitations in daily activities, night-time asthma symptoms and if 'your peak flow readings coded yellow, i.e. less than 80% of your personal best?' The five questions are each worth a point; 'no' answers score a point. The only time the *App J* user registers as having their disease 'fully under control', according to the Global Initiative for Asthma criteria, is when they answer no to all five questions. The scores are colour-coded: five points results in a green checkmark for asthma under control; scores of two through four produce a yellow checkmark, which means the user is at risk and their asthma is not well controlled; one or zero points generates a red checkmark indicating dangerous and poorly controlled asthma. The results of the 'Check' feature are displayed as a simple list, organised by date. No notification or action results from a check in the red, however; this information is kept with the user, who can respond to the app in various ways. The responsibility to act on the numbers and analytics is left up to the app user, the asthmatic.

Visualisations of peak flow performance work on the same colour-coded scheme as control assessment. This feature not only asks the user for their numeric peak flow reading, but also to log symptoms, exercise and daily cigarette consumption; for each of these three categories the user selects none, moderate or severe. (Users can select or deselect exercise and smoking registers in the 'Personal Data' screen.) App users can also enter in notes for the day. The inclusion of fields for exercise, smoking and observation vary considerably from one mAsthma app to the next. This reflects the extent to which the app relates asthma to everyday activities in place, rather than just clinical indicators such as symptoms and medication use. Yet all data inputs were restricted to binary options and drop-down menus that restrict what factors could be reported.

Unlike the 'Check' reports, which are simply a numeric rating that signifies level of control, the 'Peak Flow Readings' can be displayed on an in-app calendar, as statistics, and in a colour-coded graph. Exercise and smoking data can be displayed visually too, allowing the user to easily toggle back and forth between screens that represent peak flow readings and personal behaviours so as to see the relationship between the two. More than simply keeping track of disease indicators, compliant care apps track lifestyle factors that could be associated with asthma control. This exceeds what paper-based asthma action plans execute; mAsthma apps draw on biomedical paradigms for platform design, but also layer in additional behavioural and lifestyle data.

App J users can also unlock the 'Export Data' option for $1.00. The benefits of unlocking data include archiving and printing records of control assessment and medication use; sharing data as a PDF, CSV file or as text in an email; and to specify and delimit data for export. For compliant care apps, like *App J*, which are made by independent developers rather than development teams embedded in health organisations, the ability to share data is restricted to manual functionality; users must select information to share, and almost always through email. Even though compliant care apps fall short of connecting users or leveraging data for public or collective use, it still reinforces the model of the care team where caregivers, providers and others assisting the user with disease management can be in the data loop.

Compliant care apps also lack GPS data: There is no option or field to indicate geographical location and the design is not built to pull in data from in-app location services. Although a very thorough disease management tool in the logic of biomedicine, place and environment rarely enters into the picture of disease assembled by *App J*. Compliant care apps focus on cultivating responsible individuals who manage disease through biomedical consumption and pharmaceutical adherence: self-monitor, take medication and report control assessment in clinical contexts. This is the foundation on which all mAsthma apps are built.

Identification of risks

In my interviews with individuals working in the field of mAsthma, I identified two principle perspectives on risk. For some individuals, adherence to treatment mandates – such as taking medication as prescribed, monitoring pulmonary performance and regular visits to the doctor – were most critical factors for mitigating asthma risks. For others, there was value in visualising where and when asthma symptoms and medication use happened. All felt that increasing awareness would naturally improve risk management behaviours.

47

Interviewees saw self-tracking as increasing awareness of disease components that users might not see otherwise. Steve, a software developer who worked as a contractor, expressed surprise that the app enabled users to see problematic places and activities that may have been overlooked, even if the person had lived most of their life with the disease.

> I had a few people email in and tell me, I have had asthma for 25 years and this has helped me get it under control because I can see when things happen, or I can track my peak flow. Clearly problems from where I lived at the time or days of the week or – different things I was doing. I found that astonishing, that this little thing can help with that. Something like that I would have expected people to have a better grasp of it on their own, I guess.

Steve underestimates asthmatic experiences – the variability of the disease as well as its complexity – and how chronic conditions become embedded in identity and everyday routines in ways that make illness difficult to see separately (Charmaz, 1991). Drew, another developer, suggested that when the app showed risk patterns through self-tracking, this information could be brought to the clinic and shared with the provider to create new, more refined care practices.

> Through the course of the tracking, it can actually help narrow in on the things that trigger symptoms and then the patient can have a conversation verbally between the care partner and the patient themselves on techniques and strategies for minimizing those risks.

If the patient-user could bring a digitised record of triggers and symptoms – patterns of disease – into the clinic, there is potential to improve care with more pointed environmental control practices. Gene, a representative from a health technology company in the process of upgrading its current mAsthma app, suggested that in-app notifications coupled with habitual self-tracking could keep the asthmatic aware of their disease even in its dormancy. An asthmatic himself, Gene described the kind of care work he wanted the app to perform:

> I want an operating system that can help me manage my disease. And that operating system has to take into account the existing management systems, my asthma action plan. I want it to tell me when I'm going off track. Essentially the coach. That coaching environment, that discreet, yet aggressive reminder and the awareness of your risks is something that is important for an asthmatic.

For Gene, the app operated like a caregiver; it made the user aware of their disease, reminding them to take medication or showing the user that their asthma is uncontrolled. The asthma action plan was the key here. Uploaded into the app, the action plan was the biomedical treatment guideline that set the stage of control assessment within the app platform.

Risk calculation and communication

Part of the disease management value that mAsthma apps promise derives from predictive algorithms that are built from 'digital risk assemblages'. In such assemblages, personal disease data are entered, disassembled and then reassembled in relation to other kinds of data – public, environmental, locational, temporal, biomedical – within the context of algorithms that assess risk. As Gene told me, 'There is a multiplicity of ways to have a system use data and think. So we are really deploying algorithms to help predict when you may be at greater risk.' Most apps (*App J* served as an example) work from the asthma action plan to assess control; they do so in ways that stick to binary inputs – yes or no – and familiar colour-coded schemes. Jay described the ways in which the app did the thinking for the patient-user.

> The data is analyzed for them. I mean, I see what they see and it's not rocket science, its traffic lights. It's been simplified to the point that you can simply look at the graph and know based on – if you know traffic lights, you know how well you are doing. And so an app that requires a lot of instructions, they are getting it wrong. If it's an app, it should be intuitive. So it should be that simple.

Underlying Jay's statement was the assumption that asthma sufferers were unaware of their disease state, unaware of when their asthma was uncontrolled. However, there may be important differences between how patients assess asthma control and how it is assessed clinically. The benchmarks and indicators that patients use are not incorporated into the app design, only biomedical categories.

Some apps, those that fall into the environmental health and participatory epidemiology category, have started to bring in local environmental data. In most cases, these are merely notifications of environmental conditions rather than predictive algorithms per se. Most mAsthma project teams see value in layering environmental information into their platforms and are working to build in local valence if not operational already. Steve had a personal stake in bringing environmental data into his mAsthma app: The app project stemmed from his role as caregiver for his asthmatic son.

> That is one of the things on my big ideas list, is to find a public weather source that I can use to either say, if this is your location, this is your pollen count today. Or something like that. Or in a more predictive way – say, the pollen count is going to be X tomorrow, be prepared. Be aware of your symptoms or something like that. So it doesn't do it yet, but like I said, this matters to me because one of the triggers for my son is allergies so that kind of information would be helpful. Living where we do, I don't listen to the weather forecast everyday because it doesn't change day to day that much. So something that tells me proactively would be good....

In addition to local weather and pollen information, many development teams wanted to bring air quality alerts into apps.

> Let's say an ozone level would go up and that would lead to all of a sudden more asthma happening. Ozone was a direct relationship. As soon as the ozone went up, the asthma rates went up. The idea was, maybe we can provide a warning system for people who live in a certain area, that when ozone is going up, you can get a text message to say, listen, in your area – because we know where all these numbers are and where people are, because everything is GPS now. So we are able to make that connection. Again, this is all in real time that we have this information.

Here, reference was to air quality indicators with well-documented relationships to asthma: pollen and ozone. All interviewees suggested that push notifications could pre-emptively alert users to atmospheric conditions that might make it more difficult to breathe. Drew, who managed the mAsthma development project for his company, noted that an app's GPS function would create a facility to provide warnings about adverse environmental conditions in the app users locality:

> Ultimately the goal is to have a database of information on asthma practice and on asthma care and multiple sensor systems feeding data into that database and then based upon that database, we hope to apply an algorithm to be able to predict increasing risk to the patient. So we know that the behavior of an asthmatic is important, but we also know its not all the time the behavior, there may be external stimuli, environmental stimuli. So one of the things that

the smart phone allows us to do, is to use the GPS and that looks out at the environment and collects information about not only the person's location, but what is the environment he's in? Is there poor air quality at this time? Is the pollen count up? And then collectively, in a community way, we can look and say, by the way, ten to twenty asthmatics in your neighborhood have just taken their rescue inhalers. And you should be aware.

Most of the app developers I interviewed saw scope for using local environmental data from state or federal agencies, but some also identified the potential for crowdsourcing GPS data on user symptoms and medication use. Such crowdsourcing would add environmental health data generated by a collective public that is currently lacking in government-derived environmental information.

Risk politics

Although all interviewees in the study reported interest in GPS data on disease, a few suggested that environmental risks were not (and should not be) the primary focus of the app or the asthmatic. They argued that asthma was best addressed through treatment adherence; medication use was the risk management practice most effective for individual asthmatics. For example, Tyler noted that the app could generate clear information on adherence and this was something individuals could act on and take responsibility for; air quality could not be made accessible and controlled in the same way:

> It [information on air pollution] is certainly very good information to know from a population health standpoint, but it would be something that would be difficult for an individual to act upon. Whereas if somebody is not taking their meds, then that needs to be addressed immediately and could be addressed immediately using our tool. We have been focusing more on the behavior components and things that we can correct to get the user back on the adherence track. There might be additional improvements available from a population health standpoint, but ours is really more on an individual patient, individual transaction basis.

For Tyler, even if disease data could be geocoded and crowdsourced, environmental risks lay outside the realm of individual agency. In his view the health impacts of air pollution or high pollen counts, for example, were more effectively managed through medication regimes that provide asthmatics with a degree of biological protection. Dr Zee, who worked with one of the development teams, noted that taking medication routinely prevented disruptions to everyday activities – work and school for example – that would have to be tolerated if environmental control strategies were used to manage asthma:

> Is knowing the location that you used your Albuterol key to gaining better control of your asthma? The answer is no. Albuterol is a rescue medicine. You can use it in different places. It's not really going to make a difference. There are unusual cases where you may be sitting next to a smoker, so if you know that that is the case in that location, that may help. But that is a small portion. As a matter of fact, there really is a small portion of benefit from that. So that is not asking the right question. Asking a question like why are the asthma rates so high and why is adherence so low? What can we do about that? So that goes back to, okay, well now we have to look at the population. And really find out why is it that that is the case? After all, we know that that is causing the problem, the majority of the problem is by non-adherence and not proper management. So what can we do about that? So again, with the chronic diseases, you have to ask the right question so that you have the best possible solution to those questions.

Dr Zee thought treatment adherence was key to managing asthma risk. In his view, if an asthma sufferer took their medication as prescribed, and regularly monitored pulmonary performance, for example, then their asthma would be well controlled; there was no real need to control environmental triggers as individuals would be protected by their medication. Their location became irrelevant as the medication would protect them wherever they were. In this framing of risk, the danger stemmed from the sufferers' failure to take their medication as prescribed not from the triggers in their environment.

Discussion

There are two types of risk that could be addressed by mAsthma apps and their developers: the risk within the patient, which can be mitigated by medication, and the risk from the environment that can be mitigated by identifying and avoiding environmental triggers. As I have shown in this article, mAsthma app design emphasises the danger within the sufferer and the risk of non-adherence. The emphasis on the dangers of non-adherence aligns with biomedical mandates that address the asthma epidemic with pharmaceutical regimes; this form of risk stems from biopolitical logics where health is governed through the critique and management of individual lifestyle and behavioural choices (Dumit, 2012; Rose, 2006). While developers of these apps do recognise environmental dangers, when they are included in apps they operate in such a way as to place the focus on individual not collective action to address the danger. For example, apps are designed around individual actions rather than collective action that might address issues such as socio-economic conditions, air pollution or poor housing stock, which are associated with asthma morbidity and prevalence (Cakici & Sanches, 2014; Cheney-Lippold, 2011; Fortun et al., 2014). The apps and their developers place disease and risk data into dense information networks that privilege biomedical paradigms; this tends to leave or bracket out the emplaced knowledge and affect that anchor individuals' asthmatic care practices. The app remediates disease and risk through notifications, visual analytics and control algorithms that direct mAsthma users towards biomedical risks and management practices rather than local, emplaced, context-dependent ones (Gold & Wright, 2005; Johnson, 2014; van Loon, 2014).

Writing about virtual worlds and bodies, Boellstorff suggests that by participating and engaging with digital platforms, the user becomes emplaced; Boellstorff thinks about digital emplacement in terms of indexicality:

> When Heidegger referred to techne as making something appear 'as this or that, in this way or that way,' he emphasized an indexicality, a relation of pointing, that lies behind the mutually constitutive being of body and world. (Boellstorff, 2011, p. 514)

There is a gap between the binary code, 0 and 1, that points to the digital body; the gap between the symptom event and the yes/no checkboxes used to calculate whether the asthmatic's disease is controlled, for example. Between the virtual and actual is 'meaning-making, value production, subjectivation, and social praxis' (Boellstorff, 2011). To understand the impact of risk remediation, attention must be paid to the indexical relationship between disease in the app and disease in the material world that triggers asthma. Risks materialise in mAsthma apps and related information systems in ways that make them active agents in disease management (van Loon, 2014, p. 448). This is a different kind and order of risk than that of bodily knowledge (Latour, 2004). While some digital health technologies advance and leverage patient experiences to further disease understanding

(Sosnowy, 2014), mAsthma apps codify experiences in numerical accounts and biomedical algorithms that leave little room for user narratives. Such codification and formulaic care does little to advance understanding of patient beliefs, values and experiences, which some scholars identify as critical information for efforts that hope to improve health decision-making (Horne and Weinman 2002; Zinn, 2005). These platforms prioritise 'standardized and transportable knowledge over local and context-dependent knowledge' (Cakici & Sanches, 2004, p. 400). Location and time stamping made possible through geocoding executes a different kind of emplaced knowledge of disease. 'Places' that produce symptoms are rendered into locations, static, unitary objects that can be easily compared and circulated in databases, rather than rich environments with social actors, key landmarks, seasonal textures and biographical narratives. There is value in both modes of emplacement, but the affects will be different. mAsthma apps count on users taking action on 'invisible and abstract health risks' even though these risks have been detached from sensory experiences and perceptions (Bell, 2014, p. 166).

mAsthma apps are designed to intervene in the informal everyday world of asthma care; they work to rationalise care practices by identifying, measuring and calculating risk based on algorithms that use biomedical criteria for evaluating asthma management, such as whether a patient's illness is well controlled or poorly controlled, for example. The criteria include peak flow readings, asthmatic events and medication use, prescription refill records, and observations of daily living. They reconfigure embodied knowledge about health and illness but also remediate how to use risk knowledge. However, as Cott and Tierney point out:

> In everyday life individuals rarely adopt a formal approach to risk and uncertainty, they rarely use concrete measurements of probability as the basis for their decisions. (Cott & Tierney, 2013, p. 403; see also; Zinn, 2008)

mAsthma app users may experience 'the discursive reorganisation of their bodies' and practices as different 'regimes of meaning' structured by biomedical standards (Rich & Miah, 2014, p. 307). User data are contextualised amid expert-defined norms and government guidelines for well-controlled and poorly controlled asthma. The hope is that as the app makes visible personal disease data in relation to biomedical benchmarks, mAsthma users will be compelled towards better adherence. This logic builds on the idea that data visualisations have agentive force (Cohn, 2010; Ruckenstein, 2014, p. 73). In-app asthma action plans exemplify how biomedical standards are remediated within a self-surveillance system that directs patients to take action according to their personal risk level. Apps also 'push' responsible care in a way paper-based plans could not (Johnson, 2014; van Loon, 2014). Self-tracking platforms entice engagement through reminders and colour-coded visualisation that map users' disease data against a biomedical index. Environmental information and treatment reminders are 'pushed' through app notifications, an example of 'push responsibilisation' which places responsibility for care squarely on users, and in particular, management of risk through calculation (Johnson, 2014, p. 346.) Making 'action plans' digital, however does not automatically lead to behavioural changes; change mechanisms – such as providing instruction and 'graded tasks' – are generally not built into apps (Conroy, Yang, & Maher, 2014; Direito et al., 2014). More than merely adopting an app, users must change their own practices; apps cannot make changes for them.

Those involved in the design and development of mAsthma who I interviewed believed that increased awareness would seamlessly translate into improved disease management. Self-tracking practices, several interviewees noted, generated new modes of awareness. As Ruckenstien has argued:

> [They] make known something that is typically not a subject of reflection, with the aim of converting previously undetected bodily reactions and behavioral clues into traceable and perceptible information. (Ruckenstein, 2014, p. 69)

Self-tracking technologies, in the case of mAsthma apps, go hand in hand with data analytics designed to make bodily signs, behaviours and movements visible and legible. Embodied observations – when logged, made digital and visible in new ways – are thought to increase individual control over disease management. This is of a different order than the emplaced practices used to care for asthma without mAsthma apps. Rather than anchored in the rhythms of everyday life, local places and social relations, mAsthma apps work through digital assemblages that 'abstract and slice' users *and* places to create data doubles (Ruckenstein, 2014, p. 69).

In environmental health and participatory epidemiology apps, development teams argued that the risk of environmental exposures could be made more visible (and action-able) through collective data sourcing. App design, however, still keeps risk management at the individual level. Even when mAsthma apps signal what environments might be risky (ozone or pollen counts), it is up to the app user to take responsibility for and act to manage these risks. When asked if there was interest in the locational and environmental data that mAsthma apps could provide, several interviewees indicated that such data were not yet relevant or useful. They placed emphasis on getting adherence data and prompting patient-users to follow treatment regimes. Their perception was that those investing in apps were primarily interested in adherence, rather than local or domestic environmental conditions. Some interviewees felt that nothing could be done about the environment, which they saw as beyond the scope of care that health practitioners and case managers could provide. One interviewee stated that emphasis should be weighted towards adher-ence because that was an evidence-based means to improve patient outcomes. These views reinforce the idea that environmental management is a second-order risk manage-ment strategy (Foster & Heyman, 2013); awareness and action on environmental risks, at least in biomedical arenas, is often subsumed by the emphasis on adherence to controller medications, which must be taken daily. As long as mobile app development is tied to entrenched biomedical logics and infrastructures, these technologies will continue to exploit personal analytics for 'affect amplification' that points and pushes us towards the right things to care for (Probyn, 2004, p. 26; Rich & Miah, 2014, p. 310).

Conclusion

If emplaced care describes the ways in which asthma is addressed through embodied attention to place – surrounding environments, time of day and year, social relations and everyday routines – mAsthma apps leave out biographical, affective and ecological details important for gaining insight into how those suffering from asthma live with their disordered breathing. Such detail provides precisely the insight that risk study scholars suggest is needed for making sense of challenges in disease management (such as non-adherence). Certainly mAsthma apps emplace disease, risk and care through the very act of tracking, archiving and visualising data, but it is emplacement of a different order; one in which disease, and its associated risks and care responses are remediated in digital assemblages based on neoliberal paradigms. In mAsthma apps, personal data are tracked and analysed using biomedical logics that strip user data of context-specific detail. Such design choices are meant to reduce and make sense of the heterogeneous, multiple and variable characteristics of asthma – the messy details and undisciplined responses that make asthma so difficult to research and manage. Although limiting, extractive and abstracting, there is also potential for the algorithms and assemblages of mAsthma apps to make sense of environmental health dynamics that exceed the capacities of both the emplaced asthmatic caring for disordered breathing and biomedicine itself.

Both embedded within and an extension of chronic care infrastructures, mAsthma apps reinforce existing approaches to asthma, but also highlight components of disease, risk and care that may have been overlooked, or might have been difficult to account for. In this sense, mAsthma apps perform important epistemic work through remediation, digital ways of knowing based on a confluence of epistemes – patient, biomedical, public health and algorithmic. mAsthma apps ask users to adopt new risk management practices; yet, clearly, asthmatics are not the only users of emerging digital platforms: Researchers, clinicians, pharmaceutical companies and government agencies are invested, too. Perhaps, then, our response as critical digital health studies scholars should be: How might the design of digital health assemblages remediate a broader, collaborative politics of care?

Disclosure statement

No potential conflict of interest was reported by the author.

References

Alaszewski, A. (2013). Editorial: Vulnerability and risk across the life course. *Health, Risk, and Society, 15*(5), 381–389. doi:10.1080/13698575.2013.822852

Bell, K. (2014). Science, policy, and the rise of 'thirdhand smoke' as a public health issue. *Health, Risk & Society, 16*(2), 154–170. doi:10.1080/13698575.2014.884214

Bender, B. G., & Bender, S. E. (2005). Patient-identified barriers to asthma treatment adherence: Responses to interviews, focus groups, and questionnaires. *Immunology and Allergy Clinics of North America, 25*(1), 107–130. doi:10.1016/j.iac.2004.09.005

Boellstorff, T. (2011). Placing the virtual body: Avatar, chora, cypherg. In F. E. Mascia-Lees (Ed.), *A companion to the anthropology of the body and embodiment* (pp. 504–520). UK: Wiley-Blackwell.

Bolter, J. D., & Grusin, R. (1999). *Remediation: Understanding new media.* Cambridge, MA: MIT Press.

Boulet, L. P. (1998). Perception of the role and potential side effects of inhaled corticosteroids among asthmatic patients. *CHEST Journal, 113*(3), 587–592.

Brown, P., Mayer, B., Zavestoski, S., Luebke, T., Mandelbaum, J., & McCormick, S. (2003). The health politics of asthma: Environmental justice and collective illness experience in the United States. *Social science & medicine, 57*(3), 453–464.

Cakici, B., & Sanches, P. (2014). Detecting the visible: The discursive construction of health threats in a syndromic surveillance system design. *Societies, 4*(2), 399–413. doi:10.3390/soc4030399

Carlsson, L., & Sandström, A. (2008). Network governance of the commons. *International Journal of the Commons, 2*(1), 33–54. doi:10.18352/ijc.20

Chambre, S. M., & Goldner, M. (Eds.). (2008). *Patients, consumers, and civil society*. UK: Emerald Group Publishing Limited.

Charmaz, K. (1991). *Good days, bad days: The self and chronic illness in time*. New Brunswick: Rutgers University Press.

Cheney-Lippold, J. (2011). A new algorithmic identity: Soft biopolitics and the modulation of control. *Theory, Culture & Society, 28*(6), 164–181. doi:10.1177/0263276411424420

Cohn, S. (2010). Picturing the brain inside, revealing the illness outside: A comparison of the different meanings attributed to brain scans by scientists and patients. In J. Edwards, P. Harvey, P. Wade (Eds.), *Technologized images, technologized bodies* (pp. 65–84). New York, NY: Berghahn Books.

Conroy, D. E., Yang, C. H. & Maher, J. P. (2014). Behavior change techniques in top-ranked mobile apps for physical activity. *American Journal of Preventive Medicine, 46*(6), 649–652.

Cott, C. A., & Tierney, M. C. (2013). Acceptable and unacceptable risk: Balancing everyday risk by family members of older cognitively impaired adults who live alone. *Health, Risk & Society, 15* (5), 402–415. doi:10.1080/13698575.2013.801936

Direito, A., Dale, L. P., Shields, E., Dobson, R., Whittaker, R., & Maddison, R. (2014). Do physical activity and dietary smartphone applications incorporate evidence-based behaviour change techniques? *BMC Public Health, 14*(1), 646. doi:10.1186/1471-2458-14-646

Dumit, J. (2012). *Drugs for life: How pharmaceutical companies define our health*. Durham, NC: Duke University Press.

Fortun, M., Fortun, K., Costelloe-Kuehn, B., Saheb, T., Price, D., Kenner, A., & Crowder, J. (2014). Asthma, culture, and cultural analysis: Continuing challenges. In A. R. Brasier (Ed.), *Heterogeneity in Asthma* (pp. 321–332). New York: Springer.

Foster, J., & Heyman, B. (2013). Drinking alcohol at home and in public places and the time framing of risks. *Health, Risk, & Society, 15*(6–7), 511–524. doi:10.1080/13698575.2013.839779

Freifeld, C. C., Chunara, R., Mekaru, S. R., Chan, E. H., Kass-Hout, T., Iacucci, A. A., & Brownstein, J. S. (2010). Participatory epidemiology: Use of mobile phones for community-based health reporting. *PLoS Med, 7*(12), e1000376. doi:10.1371/journal.pmed.1000376

French, M., & Smith, G. (2013). 'Health' surveillance: New modes of monitoring bodies, popula-tions, and polities. *Critical Public Health, 23*(4), 383–392.

Gold, D. R., & Wright, R. (2005). Population disparities in asthma. *Annual Review of Public Health, 26*, 89–113. doi:10.1146/annurev.publhealth.26.021304.144528

Haggerty, K. D., & Ericson, R. V. (2000). The surveillant assemblage. *The British Journal of Sociology, 51*(4), 605–622. doi:10.1080/00071310020015280

Hodgetts, D., Chamberlain, K., Gabe, J., & Dew, K. (2011). Emplacement and everyday use of medications in domestic dwellings. *Health & Place, 17*(1), 353–360. doi:10.1016/j.healthplace.2010.11.015

Holt, M. (2013). Enacting and imagining gay men: The looping effects of behavioural HIV surveillance in Australia. *Critical Public Health, 23*(4), 404–417.

Horne, R., & Weinman, J. (2002). Self-regulation and self-management in asthma: Exploring the role of illness perceptions and treatment beliefs in explaining non-adherence to preventer medication. *Psychology & Health, 17*(1), 17–32. doi:10.1080/08870440290001502

Johnson, S. A. (2014). "Maternal devices", social media, and the self-management of pregnancy, mothering, and child health. *Societies, 4*(2), 330–350. doi:10.3390/soc4020330

Kenner, A. (2013). Caring for asthma with the Buteyko method: On how to make breath visible. In G. Mohacsi (Ed.), *Ecologies of care: Innovations through technologies, collectives, and senses*. Osaka: Osaka University.

Langstrup, H. (2013). Chronic care infrastructures and the home. *Sociology of Health & Illness, 35* (7), 1008–1022. doi:10.1111/shil.2013.35.issue-7

Latour, B. (2004). How to talk about the body? The normative dimension of science studies. *Body & Society, 10*(2–3), 205–229. doi:10.1177/1357034X04042943

Lehoux, P., Saint-Arnaud, J., & Richard, L. (2004). The use of technology at home: What patient manuals say and sell vs. what patients face and fear. *Sociology of Health & Illness, 26*(5), 617–644. doi:10.1111/shil.2004.26.issue-5

Lupton, D. (2013a). The digitally engaged patient: Self-monitoring and self-care in the digital health era. *Social Theory & Health, 11*(3), 256–270. doi:10.1057/sth.2013.10

Lupton, D. (2013b). Quantifying the body: Monitoring and measuring health in the age of mHealth technologies. *Critical Public Health*, 23(4), 393–403. doi:10.1080/09581596.2013.794931

Lupton, D. (2013c). Risk and emotion: Towards an alternative theoretical perspective. *Health, Risk & Society*, 15(8), 634–647. doi:10.1080/13698575.2013.848847

Lupton, D. (2014a). Beyond techno-utopia: Critical approaches to digital health technologies. *Societies*, 4(4), 706–711. doi:10.3390/soc4040706

Lupton, D. (2014b). Apps as artefacts: Towards a critical perspective on mobile health and medical apps. *Societies*, 4(4), 606–622. doi:10.3390/soc4040606

Lupton, D. (2016). Digital risk society. In J. Zinn, A. Burgess, & A. Alemmano (Eds.), *The Routledge handbook of risk studies*. Houndmills: Palgrave Macmillan.

Marsan, C. D. (2010, August 8). iPhone apps that could save your life. *Network World*. Retrieved from http://www.macworld.com/article/1153111/iphoneapps_lifesavers.html

Martin, A., Myers, N., & Viseu, A. (2015). The politics of care in technoscience. *Social Studies of Science*, 45(4), 625–641. doi:10.1177/0306312715602073

Mitman, G. (2007). *Breathing space: How allergies shape our lives and landscapes*. New Haven, CT: Yale University Press.

Murphy, M. (2006). *Sick building syndrome and the problem of uncertainty: Environmental politics, technoscience, and women workers*. Durham, NC: Duke University Press.

National Asthma Control Initiative. (2013, January) Putting guidelines into action. *National Heart, Lung, and Blood Institute*, Retrieved November 18, 2015, from https://www.nhlbi.nih.gov/health-pro/resources/lung/naci/discover/priorities.htm

Probyn, E. (2004). Teaching bodies: Affects in the classroom. *Body & Society*, 10, 21–43. doi:10.1177/1357034X04047854

Rand, C., Wright, R., Cabana, M. D., Foggs, M. B., Halterman, J. S., Olson, L., ... Taggart, V. (2012). Mediators of asthma outcomes. *Journal of Allergy and Clinical Immunology*, 129(3), S136–S141. doi:10.1016/j.jaci.2011.12.987

Reno, J. (2011). Beyond risk: Emplacement and the production of environmental evidence. *American Ethnologist*, 38(3), 516–530. doi:10.1111/j.1548-1425.2011.01320.x

Rich, E., & Miah, A. (2014). Understanding digital health as public pedagogy: A critical framework. *Societies*, 4(2), 296–315. doi:10.3390/soc4020296

Rose, N. (2006). *The politics of life itself: Biomedicine, power, and subjectivity in the twenty-first century*. Princeton, NJ: Princeton University Press.

Ruckenstein, M. (2014). Visualized and interacted life: Personal analytics and engagements with data doubles. *Societies*, 4(2), 68–84. doi:10.3390/soc4010068

Shapiro, N. (2015). Attuning to the chemosphere: Domestic formaldehyde, bodily reasoning, and the chemical sublime. *Cultural Anthropology*, 30(3), 368–393. doi:10.14506/ca30.3

Sosnowy, C. (2014). Practicing patienthood online: Social media, chronic illness, and lay expertise. *Societies*, 4(2), 316–329. doi:10.3390/soc4020316

Stewart, K. (2011). Atmospheric attunements. *Environment and Planning D: Society and Space*, 29(3), 445–453. doi:10.1068/d9109

The Global Asthma Network. (2014). *The global asthma report 2014*. Auckland: Global Asthma Network.

The Lancet. (2008). Asthma: Still more questions than answers. *The Lancet*, 372(9643), 1009. doi:10.1016/S0140-6736(08)61414-2

Thing, L. F., & Ottesen, L. S. (2013). Young people's perspectives on health, risks and physical activity in a Danish secondary school. *Health, Risk & Society*, 15(5), 463–477. doi:10.1080/13698575.2013.802294

Till, C. (2014). Exercise as labour: Quantified self and the transformation of exercise into labour. *Societies*, 4(2), 446–462. doi:10.3390/soc4030446

van Boven, J., Trappenburg, J., van der Molen, T., & Chavannes, N. H. (2015). Towards tailored and targeted adherence assessment to optimise asthma management. *NPJ Primary Care Respiratory Medicine*, 25, 1–6. doi:10.1038/npjpcrm.2015.46

van Loon, J. (2014). Remediating risk as matter-energy-information flows of avian influenza and BSE. *Health, Risk & Society*, 16(5), 444–458. doi:10.1080/13698575.2014.936833

Whitmarsh, I. (2008). *Biomedical ambiguity: Race, asthma, and the contested meaning of genetic research in the Caribbean*. Ithaca: Cornell University Press.

Williams, L. K., Pladevall, M., Xi, H., Peterson, E. L., Joseph, C., Lafata, J. E., ... & Johnson, C. C. (2004). Relationship between adherence to inhaled corticosteroids and poor outcomes among adults with asthma. *Journal of Allergy and Clinical Immunology, 114*(6), 1288–1293.

Zinn, J. O. (2005). The biographical approach: A better way to understand behaviour in health and illness. *Health, Risk & Society, 7*(1), 1–9. doi:10.1080/13698570500042348

Zinn, J. O. (2008). Heading into the unknown: Everyday strategies for managing risk and uncertainty. *Health, Risk & Society, 10*(5), 439–450. doi:10.1080/13698570802380891

Digital 'solutions' to unhealthy lifestyle 'problems': the construction of social and personal risks in the development of eCoaches

Samantha Adams and Maartje Niezen

Tilburg Institute of Law, Technology and Society, Tilburg University, Tilburg, The Netherlands

In this article, we critically interrogate the discourses used during the development of eCoaches. We draw on data from a four-phase qualitative study about the ethical, legal and social aspects of using digital technologies to encourage lifestyle changes that was conducted in the Netherlands between March 2014 and May 2015. The four phases of this study included interviews, document analysis, participant observation, interventionist workshops on legal issues and a forward-looking techno-ethical scenarios workshop. We use data from the first three phases to identify how both health-related and technology-related risks for individuals and society were constructed. There were multiple, concurrent references to risk in the programme and project documents, as well as in the various discussions we observed among designers. We discuss three major constructions of risk found in these discourses: risks to the health system, risks of developing an ineffective eCoach and new risks to the individual user. We argue that these three constructions feed particular norms and values into the design of the resultant eCoaches, whereby notions such as effectiveness, social solidarity, responsibility for health and individual autonomy (and thus, our understanding of what constitutes 'risk') are redefined. Understandings of risk may shift once users begin engaging with these eCoaches in practice. Future research should therefore also examine (discursive) constructions and understandings of digital risk from the perspective of the users of such technologies.

Introduction

During the last 20–30 years, in high-income countries such as the Netherlands, there has been a rapid development of eHealth technologies – web-based health environments intended to improve (self-) care for individuals and populations. With recent developments in mobile technologies, these environments have expanded to include devices such as cell phones, personal digital assistants, tablets and wearable monitors such as smart watches (collectively known as consumer mHealth). Although programmes for online coaching (eCoaching), especially for lifestyle-related processes such as weight loss or smoking cessation are not new, the increased use of consumer-targeted mobile devices and their intertwining with various aspects of daily lives has led to renewed interest in this particular area of digital health. Whereas online coaching began with digital provision of (primarily text-based) information, advances in multimedia interfaces have enabled other forms of information presentation (such as pictures and graphics) and exchange, thereby increasing possibilities for providing personalised health information to individual users of these devices. With current and future health challenges increasingly being attributed to lifestyle-related non-communicable diseases, various stakeholders seek to capitalise on the possibilities afforded by these devices for ostensibly improving individual and population health.

eCoaches use devices and sensors to gather information about individual behaviour and transform this into targeted feedback for behavioural change. By monitoring both public and personal spaces, including the human body, these technologies contribute to what Lupton (2013, 2015) calls digital surveillance, which she has argued has opened a new field of inquiry regarding the 'digital risk society', whereby what is identified as 'risky' is increasingly configured and reproduced by digital media, devices and software. Technologies act not only as mediators of risk, but often also as sources of new concepts of risk.

In this article, we seek to contribute to the discussion on 'digitised risk' (Lupton, 2013) by examining how different risk discourses are configured in the *design* and *development* of lifestyle mobile app-based eCoaches that promote 'healthy' behaviours. Viewing materialities and discourses as inextricably intertwined (Beck & Kropp, 2011), we critically interrogate the discourses used by funders, designers and developers of these apps to identify how both health-related and technology-related risks are constructed and subsequently feed particular norms and values into the design of the resultant eCoaches.

Discursively constructing health risks and using digital technologies to govern behaviour

While there are multiple theories on risk, scholars in sociology generally identify three major perspectives: the risk society perspective, the cultural/symbolic perspective and the governmentality perspective (see, for example, Adam & van Loon, 2000; Beck, 1992; Douglas, 1990; Douglas & Wildavsky, 1983; Lupton, 1999, 2006a). In this article, we draw on the governmentality perspective that is grounded in Foucault's work on historical shifts in social/political power relations as states grappled with retaining control over populations (Foucault, 1991; Rose, O'Malley, & Valverde, 2006). Scholars working from this perspective tend to examine how mechanisms of governance attempt to realise political programmes or social goals by exerting power at the level of individual behaviour. Using instruments such as counting, assessment, categorisation and judging/disciplining (Dean, 2000; Taylor-Gooby, 2008) places emphasis on measuring risk assessment, perception and evaluation at both the individual and societal level, and identifying those persons both *at* risk and *posing* a risk, whereby how risks are defined can serve to alter or maintain the power structure of a given society (Lupton, 1993, 2006a, 2006b).

Central to this approach is the recognition of the constructed nature of risks, whereby the notion refers to the consequences of what *might* happen following specific choices made in particular circumstances. Given specific focus on *possibilities* for averting/ avoiding danger, constructions of risk are based on *predictions* about behaviour distribution and possible effects of transgression across populations (Taylor-Gooby, 2008). Moreover, risk is often used to refer to the possibility of damage, whereby what is at stake is of value to at least *some* persons (Van Asselt & Renn, 2011). Risk construction is largely a discursive practice that problematises certain phenomena in particular socio-cultural contexts and enables implementation of specific governance programmes. This is reflected, for example, in discourses arguing the benefits of 'good health' for both individuals and society that are used to steer personal choices and behaviours. Representations of possible health-related risks found in policy documents or promotional items serve to advance an agenda that is centred on classical health promotion strategies and encourages specific forms of individual and collective action (Hooker, Carter, & Davey, 2009; Lupton, 1993; Singleton, 2005). Such representations frame risks not only in the negative (what might happen, such as possible detrimental effects), but also communicate positive benefits (possibilities for averting danger, such as the number of lives saved) of complying with a given strategy or policy (Hooker et al., 2009).

Understandings of risks to personal health are further influenced by the available technologies and methods for developing knowledge about health. What constitutes 'good' health-related behaviour (and who is responsible for it) fluctuates in relation to technological momentum (Adams & de Bont, 2007; Beck-Gersheim, 2000; Hooker et al., 2009). The newest iteration is found in the mHealth apps made available on smart phones and in sensors with related software that offer new ways of monitoring and measuring the human body (Lupton, 2012, 2013). With these technologies, the body is opened up to an external gaze that provides access to reflective health or medical information about the individual. While this information is promoted as helping the individual user understand his/her health, it can also be used by others to identify risky behaviours and/or at-risk individuals.

With new technologies, identifying probable health risks is based on algorithmic calculations, for example, via big data analytics, which provide a scientific (and arguably more reliable) estimation of risks (Lupton, 2006b). This calculative approach to risk identification fits the paradigms of individualised and personalised health, where health risks are considered to be manageable and controllable via self-monitoring and self-care based on personalised treatments and coaching. As Lupton has argued: 'Digital technologies have become increasingly used as a tool for public health to identify "at risk" individuals and groups' (2013, p. 14). mHealth technologies seem particularly to facilitate this turn towards personalised health by catering to individual characteristics and bodily markers (Dickenson, 2013). The increased use of such technologies thus allows for digitising health risks, with eCoaches, for example, working on the premise that especially lifestyle-related health risks can be defined before they even manifest and then mitigated through self-control and discipline.

Policies for public health promotion have suggested that mitigating or averting lifestyle-related health risks may lead to improved health outcomes and cost reduction, making health in this context simultaneously an individual task, meaningful social practice and a moral responsibility (Brown, 2013; Crawford, 2006; Singleton, 2005). 'Good' health is discursively constructed as a shared socio-cultural value and an attainable goal to which all individuals can and should aspire, evidenced in measures taken to reduce risks to their personal health, such as the appropriation of information technologies (Harris, Wyatt, & Wathen, 2010). However, encouraging individuals to follow proposed strategies for a greater social good may conflict in practice with other modern social values, including individual choice and autonomy. While there is possibility for users to resist prescribed 'good' behaviours, such as informed consumerism (Felt, Bister, Strassnig, & Wagner, 2009), this is largely discouraged in the name of good citizenship. Beck-Gersheim (2000) therefore refers to public health policies as voluntary compulsion. Singleton (2005) similarly argues that participation in programmes that govern personal and public health becomes simultaneously optional and obligatory.

For this reason, we are interested in teasing out how risks to 'good' health as constructed in the current Dutch health landscape are purportedly 'resolved' or 'combated' by the uptake of specific technologies, such as the mobile application-based eCoach. We follow the development of two eCoaches in order to understand how these applications become imbued with certain norms and values, such as the moral imperative to be responsible for one's health.

Methods

In this article, we draw on data from the 'Socially Robust eCoaching' project, a one-year project on the ethical, legal and social (ELSA) aspects of using digital technologies to encourage 'healthy' lifestyle changes.

Context In 2011, a public–private partnership comprising Philips Research, the Dutch National Brain & Cognition Initiative and Technology Foundation 'STW' established a five-year, nationally-funded research programme, 'Healthy Lifestyle Solutions.' Five research teams are developing projects focused on: combining established face-to-face coaching techniques with (new) digital technologies, providing personalised, daily feedback and encouraging healthy behaviours related to exercise, diet, sleep patterns and stress reduction (STW Website, 2011). Following initial programme meetings that revealed ethical concerns about continuously monitoring individuals and using persuasive strategies for behavioural change, in 2013 the Healthy Lifestyle Solutions programme issued a call for proposals for an additional, one-year research project on social, legal and ethical aspects of eCoaching to make the programme more 'socially robust', which resulted in the Socially Robust eCoaching project that produced the data used in this article.

Data Collection The Socially Robust eCoaching project comprised four phases of qualitative research. Phase 1 used a literature and web review to formulate the ELSA framework, followed by document analysis and telephone interviews with project leaders for all projects. Of these projects, two were selected for deeper case study research.

During Phase 2, researchers conducted case study research by observing team meetings over a 2–3 month period ($n = 10–12$ per case), reviewing internal documents and conducting interviews, which allowed them to follow the development of two eCoaching apps. The researchers also held a two-hour workshop with each project team, whereby a legal scholar used a series of interactive exercises to identify the legal issues related to their respective eCoach. Observations were written in field notes (Bernard, 1994) and the workshops were recorded with permission and transcribed verbatim.

Data from the first two phases were used to develop techno-ethical scenarios in Phase 3. Technical-ethical scenarios are fictional narratives of possible future ethical controversies that provide a tool for anticipating interactions between new technologies and society and exploring the role that normative perspectives or moral values play in these interactions (Boenink, Swierstra, & Stemerding, 2010; Lucivero, 2013; Swierstra, Stemerding, & Boenink, 2009). Scenarios were developed following Boenink et al. (2010): gleaning field notes for dichotomous distinctions made by developers and listing these without exclusion or ranking, then categorising distinctions and noting potential tensions. Distinctions ranged from technical or practical (such as iPhone Operating System versus Android steering system, programming messages in English versus Dutch), to more socially oriented (willingness versus non-willingness to change, perceived versus actual behaviour) and medically specific terms (adherence versus nonadherence). Coupling these on the framework developed in phase one resulted in two scenarios, each of which began with a description of the current moral landscape in relation to lifestyle and mobile health applications, followed by a short-term scenario (2014–2019) and a long-term scenario (2020–2025).

Ten respondents from four different projects and three programme representatives participated in the workshop. To increase the spontaneity of answers and ensure that members of the same development team did not coordinate their answers, participants did not receive the scenarios ahead of time, but were given time to read them during the workshop. Following traditional focus group methodology (Krueger & Casey, 2000), respondents were asked to write their initial reactions individually. These reactions were then discussed in a plenary manner. Maartje Niezen (the second author) led the discussion and Samantha Adams (the first author) noted the answers on a flip chart. The workshop was recorded and transcribed verbatim and the flip chart pages were preserved.

Phase 4 comprised semi-structured telephone interviews ($n = 9$) with relevant stake-holders from five European countries to validate the findings from an international perspective. Because only data from the first three phases is used in this article (documents, interviews, observations and workshop), we do not further address these interviews here, but note that they revealed no new insights, indicating that saturation through methodological and data triangulation was reached (Creswell, 1998; Green & Thorogood, 2004).

Data Analysis We conducted cyclical analysis through all four phases of the study. The authors independently coded the initial workshop and observation data, first through open (inductive) coding and subsequently through deductive and axial coding (Strauss & Corbin, 1990). This enabled them to compare findings with the ELSA framework that had been defined earlier in the study and cluster the open codes into themes. Each researcher made an independent topic list and then these were compared. The identified themes and codes were similar, with only small deviations. These deviations were discussed to determine uniform terminology for a coding scheme that was then used to (re-)code all data from the project.

Although this was an independent research project, it was funded by the aforementioned public–private partnership, which arguably had varied interests in the results of this project. We therefore ensured our independent position by incorporating user committees, validation interviews and both external and internal academic peer review of our analysis and interpretation of the gathered data.

For the document, interview, observational and workshop data presented here, quotes were translated from Dutch to English by Samantha Adams (the first author, a native English speaker with certified Dutch fluency) and checked by Maartje Niezen (the second author, a native Dutch speaker) for proper capture of diction and nuance. Given the small-scale nature of the study and internal programme agreements, we use numbers to refer to respondents and refrain from providing additional contextual information. This is to protect against inferences regarding identity based on presumed gender or role in the project. Where we mention developers or designers in a collective fashion, this refers to the multidisciplinary research teams (computer scientists and medical content experts) working on the two eCoaches.

Findings

From our analysis of the data collected in the first three phases, we were able to identify in participants' statements and discussions three types of risk that they were concerned about:

- risks to the health system (and thus society at large);
- the risk of developing an ineffective solution for combating the problems identified under the first point;
- the risk to personal values introduced through the development (and use) of new technologies as solutions to these problems.

As our analysis shows, each social construct contains a discursive, behavioural and material interplay, at once both positive and negative, between social norms, individual user capabilities and technological mediation.

A health system at risk

The first risk that we identified in our analysis was the threat posed *to* the *health system* (and thus society at large) *by* the *unhealthy behaviours of individuals*. For example, the title of the programme Healthy Lifestyle *Solutions* implied that (normatively defined) 'unhealthy' lifestyle behaviours, such as lack of exercise, too much stress, certain eating habits or lack of sleep were framed as *problems*. Additionally, the 2011 project plan that led to the eCoaching programme included the following statement:

> It is expected that the number of people with chronic disease will increase dramatically in the coming years. … Some chronic diseases have been found to be linked to *unhealthy lifestyles*, such as unhealthy eating habits, physical inactivity and stressful lives.

> - During the last decade, there has been an *alarming* increase in obesity prevalence among adults and teens throughout the world, due to convenient lifestyle habits of high-fat diet and lack of exercise. Obesity has been found to increase the risk of developing diabetes, cardiovascular diseases and some cancers.
> - It is estimated that between 10 and 20% of people chronically experience sleep problems. A lack of sleep is *detrimental* [to] one's health. The functioning of the immune system is reduced while one's stress level increases.

> It is important from a societal and individual perspective that people obtain solutions that help them achieve a healthy lifestyle (emphases added).

These points framed unhealthy lifestyles as a 'problem' that threatens national (Dutch) well–being and systems that promote collective action to help individuals adopt healthy lifestyles as the 'solution' to this problem. The excerpt also stressed the urgency of taking action by using words such as *alarming* increase in specific social groups at a much greater (global) scale. This was reflected in the resulting research proposals that discussed how 'sleep deficits are reaching epidemic proportions' (Research Proposal Project 4) or highlighted 'an urgent need for (cost-)effective solutions to failed attempts to lose weight' (Research Proposal Project 5).

The programme representatives and team members of these projects embraced the idea that unhealthy lifestyles or behaviours are a major threat that needed to be addressed. For example, during the technical-ethical scenarios workshop, Respondent 4 raised the following point:

> Yesterday I read that the WHO published a report in 2014 regarding non-communicable diseases. They've formulated a number of goals regarding healthy behaviour...no, health

goals that are related to healthy behaviour. At any rate, preventing further increase in rates of obesity and decreasing the number of cardio-pulmonary illnesses.

Respondent 4's reference to such international statements is one example of how other actors take up specific discourses to advance their own goals. In the Netherlands, this is also reflected in a long-standing debate about social solidarity and the sustainability of healthcare within the social welfare state. Policymakers emphasise the collective benefits of a healthy society and health promotion discourses increasingly, which include the additional potential social (and economic) benefits of technological developments such as eCoaching. Such arguments from a societal perspective are explicit in the various programme texts and project proposals. Not only did these documents highlight collective benefits such as the collective gain in overall health and the collective reduction in health-related expenditures, but they also categorised 'unhealthy' lifestyles and behaviours, broadly defined as a risk to solidarity in that they endangered the sustainability of the health system.

The solution to this risk was then arguably found in pinpointing groups for which digital coaching interventions might curb the unhealthy behaviours before they result in poor health or disease. For example, the call for proposals issued in 2013 stated the following:

> The aim of the Healthy Lifestyle Solutions programme is to develop know-how and solutions for empowering people to adopt a lifestyle that promotes good health. ... The target population is early stage: people at risk of developing chronic medical conditions, together with people that have the aspiration to live a healthy life and would like to be supported in this.

Thus, the documents and participants depicted which types of individuals were at risk and needed the specific forms of support that the state (together with industry partners and sector professionals) could provide in order to prevent health problems before they became evident (and difficult to treat). eCoaching delivered via mobile technologies could potentially support them in a positive way, especially if they were interested in changing their behaviours but did not know how, had 'failed' in the past (Notes Programme Meeting 2013) or might 'slack off and slide into usual routines' (Research Proposal Project 4).

Developers seemed to make the (implicit) assumption that the decision to seek a coach would come from someone's personal (intrinsic) motivation to improve their health and that the eCoach would serve as additional (extrinsic) motivation to help them meet that end. They conceived of coaching techniques delivered via mobile technologies that could increase incrementally over a period of time; for example, one document suggested that, 'The coach will be the first contact in a stepped care system' (Research Proposal Project 2).

Underpinning these discussions of collective risks to the healthcare system were concerns about the *social group* (target population) for which the intervention is developed, the implied unhealthy *behaviour* and the *timing* of the intervention. Developers recognised that the technique was not failsafe: even if it reached the right group of people, it might not address the right 'unhealthy' behaviours. As the first call for projects noted, 'Part of the challenge is to observe the behaviour of coachees and classify those behaviours as desired or undesired, as healthy or unhealthy'. Moreover, if the timing was not right, the intervention would come too late to prevent the development of certain health conditions and related demands on healthcare. This latter issue reflects a progressive move towards increasingly earlier intervention in individual health practices to pre-empt specific outcomes and prevent their (negative) effects.

An interesting aspect of one of the eCoaches-in-development was the intent not only to coach individuals, but to enrol others from (online) social networks and use social media to coach each person in relation to peers. This was partially based on early internal research outcomes that suggest social support is more important than personality traits, but was also considered to be a low-threshold approach to encouraging activity among larger groups (Observation Project 1 14 July 2014), without having to deal with barriers of time and distance. It was thus also considered to increase solidarity and shared responsibility for health. The general programme text in the first call identified the challenges of social interaction as such:

> The social relation between coach and coachee that can be impoverished due to geographical distance and time restrictions is envisioned to be enhanced by increased personalisation and situational awareness. Unobtrusive monitoring of the coachee's behaviour and other bodily signals in context should contribute to a thorough understanding of the coachee's situation and facilitate creation of a sincere feeling of being understood and thoughtfully guided.

The various texts and discussions suggested that a possible breakdown of social solidarity due to the increasing demand for healthcare could be addressed by technology such as eCoaching that not only helped persons deal with their individual lifestyle and health issues but also brought people together through social networks and across perceived barriers of time and space creating solidarity in and through networks.

Calculating risk and the risk of ineffective coaching

The second risk that we identified in our analysis was the risk *developers felt* of developing an *ineffective intervention* that missed the target for a 'Healthy Lifestyle Solution'. During the Legal Workshop organised by the researchers for project 1 (see methods, data collection and Phase 2), the developers discussed the issue of effectiveness. The risk of being ineffective was partially attributed to what was *asked of the user* (that is, whether users have the right know-how and skill to input the right type of data at the right place and the right time, to ensure valid input) and partially to what was *programmed into the eCoach* (that is, the correctness of the underlying algorithm correct and its ability to generate the right advice based on input data that was adequately tailored to the needs of the individuals user). On the STW Website (2011), this was articulated in the following way:

> It will require new developments in technology, such as new network and sensor technologies that will deliver the necessary data to the automated coaching programme so that it can provide coaching and guidance. (STW Website, 2011)

Developers involved in this particular aspect of the eCoaches-in-development made a distinction between 'objective' measurement and 'subjective' experience, arguing that a combination of the two was felt to be necessary in order to generate the level of personalisation that was deemed necessary to be effective. During the technical-ethical scenario workshop, Respondent 9 said:

> The app is very dependent upon what the person logs, so I wrote down that the users should provide honest logs about their activities and weight. Maybe that can one day be

resolved with sensors – that you really know what it is... but for now it remains an important point.

Respondent 6 agreed:

These applications only have effects – positive effects – if people use them in a responsible manner. So, the more you have to assume that people use the apps well, the more dependent the effectiveness of your app or device is on how they behave.

Developers wrestled with the challenge of operationalising national norms within the technical algorithms to generate personalised advice. They felt they could not ask individuals directly whether they adhered to a given norm, as this would require users to be familiar with such norms. They were also concerned that people would either overestimate or underestimate their situation, which would result in invalid input values and potentially generate the wrong advice (Observation Project 1 14 July 2014). This led to many discussions regarding how to ensure that both the 'correctness' of the algorithm ('objective' data) and the personal experience ('subjective' data) were guaranteed in the measures taken.

Developers in Project 1 sought to resolve this dilemma by asking users for their experiences and estimates and at the same time taking an 'objective' measure through a wearable sensory device that interacted with the eCoach (Observation 18 August 2014). The eCoach was programmed to interpret this data in relation to the norm in question and generate a response that advised a particular behaviour, motivated users towards a short-term goal and provided information about the norm in order to sustain effects over a longer period of time. While one project specifically referred to techniques of persuasion (Research Proposal Project 2), researchers in Project 1 noted that it was not only about persuasion, but also fostering personal reflexivity about lived experience (Observation 18 December 2014).

In Project 2, the solution to this dilemma was sought in data analysis and the constraint-based approach (the eCoach was programmed to detect violations and generate dialogue action). Asserting that the user, not the eCoaching application, resolved the user's problem, the developers created an app that provided a 'mirror' that makes the behavioural issue evident to the user, then aided the user in tackling this problem using the eCoach (Observation 28 October 2014). Initially, Project 2 also aimed for including sensors to confirm users' input (non-obtrusive sensory measurement enables the obtainment of objective sleep data); however, this was not possible for practical reasons. The team focused instead on the possibility of testing and increasing the reliability of user input, including reflecting on how data was saved in the application.

The combination of techniques used for data input and generating advice took on the voluntary–compulsory/optional–obligatory nature that is familiar in health promotion (see section on Discursively Constructing Health Risks and Using Digital Technologies to Govern Behaviour). Users were given options from which they could choose, but information was presented such that it led to 'desirable' health-related behaviours and attitudes. That is, the choices provided by the eCoach were based on creating adherence to medical norms, under the guise of helping people recognise 'deficits' in their behaviour and learn to reflect on and correct them.

Developers were also concerned that the app would not be effective if the advice generated by the eCoach was not *tailored* well enough to fit the needs of each individual. Personalisation was one of the key tenets of the research programme, as stated in the project plan/first call for proposals:

Personalised intervention to strengthen healthy functions is a central point in both the NIBC and the NWO 2011–2014 strategy documents.

Many digital self-help programmes target large user groups and fail to take users' individual characteristics into account. The personalisation potential of mobile technologies (through the combination of computational ability, user input and – if connected – sensor-based monitoring), should ensure there is more attention to both personalised information and individual users' environmental factors. However, developers wrestled with finding the optimal mix between generic messages (did you know…), generic messages written with a tailored feel (try taking the stairs to your third-floor office today) and messages specific to a given person 'just in time and place', such as praise for achieving a specific goal (Observation Project 1 14 July 2014; 23 October 2014).

There was concern in both projects that users would quickly grow bored with receiving the same or similar messages, or the pattern of sending (e.g. at same time each day). As one of the developers from Project 2 observed during a regular project meeting:

> You want to give feedback to someone who always chooses the longest possible amount of sleeping time. But if they don't change their behaviour, then don't keep giving the same feedback. (Observation 20 September 2014)

In Project 1, developers felt that the eCoach needed to be an 'innovative' technology. Because they were targeting young adults, part of the design focused on creating a 'hip' or 'cool' gadget that individuals would want to use and encourage others to use. The nature and delivery of messages was not only about effective timing and appropriate content, but also about broadening the reach of the eCoach to more users.

Developers in Project 2 focused on 'personalisation via negotiation', which allowed the user to set goals that deviated (within certain limits) from the eCoach's suggestions and to personalise exercise time schemes. An internal document from this project stated that:

> [N]egotiation between coach and coachee about therapy properties is applied as a persuasive strategy to achieve a mutual state of commitment towards the performed exercises. (Internal document 4 June 2014)

The developers had difficulty in finding a balance between persuading the user to adhere to the optimal therapy (the calculated scheme) and allowing the user to deviate. Either too much leeway or too much steering risked diminishing the effectiveness of the therapy. Such negotiation resulted in an eCoach that provided advice with limited options, though as one developer pointed out, this meant finding the right way of phrasing the user's options was crucial:

> It is difficult to find the right words, simple so everyone can understand, but also that it exactly pinpoints what you mean, and to phrase it within the margins of the mobile screens. (Observation 10 June 2014)

The developers felt that it was crucial that users understand why particular constraints were built into the programme and receive information on the most effective course of action. In their opinion, this would enhance users' adherence to therapy and minimise their feelings of being patronised. This was evident in their discussions about how the eCoach should respond to user input, for example, in the following suggested response:

> You proposed working toward not spending more than six and a half hours in bed each day. Because limiting bed time hours is a powerful tool if you use it well, I am going to propose a different option.

At the same time, this 'personalisation via negotiation' took place within predefined parameters, meaning that the negotiating 'partners' are not necessarily equal. The constraints embedded in the system shaped the type of recommendation and dialogue taking place. The developers could personalise feedback and recommendations in terms of calculated duration, start and end of exercise but not in terms of the phrasing or ordering of generic messages, which have to have the same formats regardless of the user's characteristics. By stimulating interaction and dialogue between the eCoach and the coachee, developers believed they could set desirable targets for the individual, yet still steer behaviour to be within established norms for an effective eCoaching programme.

The idea of 'just in time and place' also raised the issue of the correct moment that the eCoach should intervene and with what type of message. Both projects followed Fogg's (2002) persuasive technologies theory, which showed a relationship between ability and motivation: when motivating users to sustain their programme, timing of recommendations is essential. Project 1 wrestled with when to benchmark and when to intervene. During a regular meeting, one of the developers questioned:

> If you try to motivate someone over the course of one week, what is the risk that they will stay in that phase of the system? The module to increase motivation is crucial, which is where the combination of tailoring and general information on the benefits comes in. (Observation 23 October 2014)

This was a recurring theme that came up again several weeks later, 'Is an evaluation halfway a good idea?' (Observation 18 December 2014)

The developers in Project 2 assumed that people would feel better just after finishing an exercise and that this was the best time to recommend starting the next exercise or propose a higher level of exercise than the one just conducted.

> Even if you feel bad and choose a shorter exercise, it is good because it personalises the app. (Observations 10 June 2014)

Developers expected users to make their own decisions, which meant that even if they altered their exercise level after an eCoach notification, developers argued that it was the user (and not the eCoach) that made the decision. However, deviation from the prescribed regime required more user effort than adhering to it. The eCoach automatically resets to the new recommended regime, which is made visible in the eCoach through a dial that is set at a default level but can be turned forward or backward according to the preferences of the individual. If users want to disregard this new setting they must undertake two actions, whereby deviation requires more conscious decision and effort than following suggested actions.

Developers recognised the need to be transparent about why certain aspects within the eCoaching programme were or were not communicated. (Observation Project 2 2 September 2014) Although they preferred not to have to explain or justify the rationale behind every aspect of the eCoach, they nonetheless recognised the need for expectation management and transparency because these factors in the design of the application needed to be tested in order to support claims regarding its effectiveness.

They were also concerned about how well the eCoach would align with the individual's daily routine and be accepted in the first place. For example, the initial call stated that:

> The motto for e-coaching is 'measure, monitor and motivate'. It is important that the individual does not find the e-coaching method to be a burden and it has to be completely acceptable on an ethical level.

The Healthy Lifestyle Solutions programme encouraged designing applications that would not be too cumbersome and intrude upon an individual's daily routine, which could result in users stopping their use. The specification for the programme identifies 'unobtrusiveness' as a key characteristic of the application or device. However, unobtrusiveness is not a static attribute, but rather, a relational property in terms of experiences and expectations, that is constructed in the interaction between a technology and its users. Because intentionally designing an 'unobtrusive' technology meant it could easily overstep the line of legitimate action in monitoring individual behaviour, designers sought a model that enabled the technology to do its work, without giving users the feeling of infringement upon their daily lives. This points to a number of ethical issues that are further discussed in the next section.

New risks to the individual

The third risk that we identified in our analysis was posed *by the technology to the individual* using the coaching app. The participants in our study formulated this kind of risk in terms of autonomy, privacy, responsibility or another *ethical issue/moral value* (not always specified) to the user of the technology. The second call for research proposals (when the programme commissioned additional research on the ELSA of eCoaching) articulated this type of risk in the following way:

> Coaching solutions collect a wealth of information about their coachees. In particular, unobtrusive, longitudinal monitoring can give rise to all kinds of acceptance issues and ethical concerns. Continuous monitoring can give rise to a feeling of 'big brother is watching you' and, even unintentionally, intimate information may be acquired. Therefore, long-term monitoring needs to be organised in such a way that it is acceptable to the individual as well as to society at large. eCoaching solutions should operate in a manner that is ethically responsible and acceptable for envisioned users.

In the technical-ethical scenario workshop, the participants discussed the extent to which automated coaches impacted on individual *autonomy* and, in turn, society. They suggested that an individual user's freedom to make his or her own choices might be hampered by the technology's ability to take over their motivation. Furthermore, the automation of user behaviour via the eCoach might affect both an individual's awareness of what is happening and the behavioural aspect of adherence. Although adherence is important with respect to effectiveness, the question remained whether use of the eCoach allowed the user to make wiser decisions or softly steers him or her through persuasive techniques into behaviours considered better by others.

In practice, these debates led to struggles over how to translate autonomy and intrinsic motivation into programming choices. The choice to increase or maintain a healthy lifestyle could be facilitated via the eCoach, yet users might feel hampered by the choices offered. Despite personalisation through negotiation, Project 2's eCoach-in-development left little room for user-initiated dialogue or actions. This was evident in the following discussion during one of the team meetings:

> *Team Member 1*: Removing, can you actually remove something? Can you explain as a user that you do not agree with something? If you do not agree, will the coach talk to you?
> *Team Member 2*: The constraint-based approach of the eCoach means that youcannot talk with your eCoach about you not wanting to do something. Youcan actually not do the exercise, but you cannot state that you do not want to do this. (Observation 17 June 2014)

One week later, the designers continued this discussion and argued that users should not be allowed too much freedom (Observation 24 June 2014). For example, they argued that if the eCoach provided a facility to defer an activity, for example, by allowing the user to perform a particular task on another day, then this might result in the subsequent accumulation of tasks, leading to nonadherence over a longer term. Thus, they agreed that the eCoach should only permit rescheduling a task, such as evaluations or exercises, for another moment on the same day that it was scheduled, in order to increase adherence and effectiveness. They argued that building in user autonomy as freedom to make their choices would not necessarily contribute to the user's desired targets.

Designers were also concerned about the *responsibility* the eCoach had towards the coachees, explicating the difference between automated and face-to-face coaching. Although eCoach developers wanted people to follow the prescribed programme, they did not want to create dangers for users or their environment. Reaching more people without the constraints of time and distance also meant the trade-off of fewer face-to-face encounters. In regular therapy, a coach can warn about specific types of risks related to the programme and regularly evaluate how the coachee is feeling. However, developers doubted the ability of the eCoach to reach this same level of responsiveness using automated algorithms, even with the best programming, and therefore questioned whether (and to what extent) the eCoach or the user was responsible for avoiding such unwanted effects.

Although the eCoach generated different types of advice, including, in some cases, when to see a physician or stop using a certain technique, developers still placed responsibility on the individual user to determine when and how use of the application was appropriate to his or her situation. This led to the interesting paradox that while users were expected to follow the advice of the eCoach in the interest of compliance and effectiveness, whereby the designers limited the number of available choices, they were also seen as responsible for their own safety and that of others. This meant that they were simultaneously expected to follow the prescribed actions and question them when necessary.

As we have already noted, the programme text steered designers towards making the eCoach as unobtrusive as possible. This design goal implies a potential trade-off with individual *privacy*. eCoaches are designed to collect and store large amounts of personal and contextual data about users. Designers were aware that users had little control over what data they supplied and how this was, in turn, used in the development of coaching messages that steer their behaviour. For example, one of the developers in Project 1 noted:

Is it possible to look for other active members and invite friends from their social network – or would this lead to some sort of social information imbalance... I know about your activity but you don't know about mine? And is there an active switch to turn off when you don't want others to see? Or should it be less personal and more anonymous – you are friend 3? (Observation 14 July 2014)

Designers noted that failing to reflect upon potential personal risks related to unobtrusive data collection, processing and distribution by the eCoach might leave such risk deliberately unconstructed in favour of avoiding 'unhealthy' behaviours.

Discussion

In this article, we have examined how the development of eCoaches embeds discursive constructions of risk at both the individual and societal levels. This case shows how organisations in the Netherlands follow (and use as justification) the larger trend already recognised in sociology (see inter alia, Lupton, 1993; Singleton, 2005) of defining specific lifestyle choices as risky behaviours that potentially lead to development of certain diseases, but can, and should, be combated using tools and programmes made available by governments, health providers and, increasingly, third parties. Funders of the Healthy Lifestyle Solutions programme framed behaviours such as poor diet, lack of exercise and sleep deprivation as problems for which and the individual project teams could develop information technology-based solutions such as eCoaches that people could be both intrinsically and extrinsically motivated to use.

We identified multiple, concurrent references to risk in the programme and project documents, and the various discussions we observed among designers. The sources depicted individuals as being both 'at risk' of sustaining or resuming bad health habits and (thereby) 'posing a risk', through their 'unhealthy' behaviour, to the sustainability of the health system and, in turn, to social solidarity. But the documents and discussions also included references to risk that are specifically attributed to the digital technologies and these particular notions of risk may be only indirectly related to health: 'calculating risk', where 'lack of personalisation of information fed back to the user' is seen as a risk to the effectiveness of the application and the underlying goals of the programme. Individual users might also 'be at risk' of infringement on privacy or autonomy, whereby the very notion of being at risk is not only about (un)healthy behaviours or lifestyle choices, but also about relational aspects of the use of technologies such as an eCoach under the guise of personal responsibility.

Under the guise of personal improvement through coaching, potentially 'at risk' (in terms of health) individuals are encouraged to interact with an automated programme, whereby they become enrolled, together with the technology, in a complex heterogeneous network of actors who have diverse interests in the outcomes (Lupton, 2015). Because the various understandings of risk lead to embeddedness of specific norms and values embedded in these socio-technical networks, the concerns of Beck-Gersheim (2000) and Singleton (2005) regarding the voluntary–compulsory, optional–obligatory nature of public health programmes become especially relevant here.

Programmes for improving health have implications for individual autonomy. Interacting with an automated programme such as an eCoach involves (partially) delegating decisions and willpower to the technology. While the designers of the eCoach emphasise its benign objective, that is enabling individuals live healthier lifestyles, they acknowledge less benign aspects; users have to give up a degree of autonomy in terms of relying on the eCoach for its reflections on their behaviour and selection of goals and acting on its advice and following its recommended changes. Users retain their 'autonomy' to act in accordance with a prescribed set of norms. Rather than demonstrating 'reflexivity' as the developers suggest, we argue that this delegation of willpower to digital technologies is likely to *decrease* human capacity to make autonomous choices in the long run, especially if the core values of transparency and opt-out options are not properly built into these (or other) digital health technologies.

Such technology may also undermine individuals' autonomy in other ways. Beyond concerns about adherence, effectiveness and achieving long-term goals, eCoaches also embed understandings of risk as a fear that those who are already disadvantaged will suffer more (Douglas, 1990). In the Dutch health policy context, this is explicitly linked to the notion of solidarity: individuals engaging in unhealthy lifestyles potentially endanger the sustainability of the health system (and thus access and benefit for others) because they tend to consume more 'health goods' than is affordable over the longer term. In identifying individuals posing a risk to the system, those behaviours classified as 'undesirable' or 'unhealthy' tend to be framed as a break-down of self-regulation that could and should be corrected in a non-burdensome way. However, there has been little attention for the possibility that the political response of stimulating technological solutions such as consumer mHealth in order to distribute responsibility for health and promote a healthy lifestyle might actually deepen existing social divides. Hence, it raises the issue of inequalities invoked by stimuli towards incorporating more digital technologies in health promotion programmes.

Mobile app-based eCoaches reflect a possible progression from behavioural steering through established persuasive coaching techniques to unprecedented levels of behavioural monitoring (Lupton, 2015). Although we did not discuss them in depth in this article, two projects were less focused on designing an actual eCoach addressing instead issues related to cognition and intentions. These projects showed a move towards developing technologies focused on *automated cognitive restructuring*, which in some cases could make automated programmes capable (through constant monitoring of thoughts/ intentions) of intervening to *prevent* undesirable behaviours. This meant that the persuasive techniques embedded in the eCoaches introduce new identifications of risky behaviour as related to 'bad' intentions.

Moreover, when such persuasive strategies are combined with real-time data being generated by different sensors, *the point of intervention* in people's daily lives *shifts* to increasingly earlier points. The algorithms and calculations thus not only allow for defining potential health risks before they manifest, but also allow for 'rewriting' human behaviour so that it fits the social norms of healthy living as a precautionary measure. Because social norms are rapidly changing, this implies that eCoaches may come to invoke measures against predicted and probable risks before it is known whether they should be regarded as harmful in the first place.

Conclusion

The wide distribution of digital consumer technologies such as smart phones has led policymakers to encourage appropriation and use of these technologies (and their associated networked apparatuses) for public health promotion. Increasingly, they also urge non-traditional actors such as small-to-medium enterprises or mobile health start-ups to help identify possible 'risk groups' for whom mobile app-based 'solutions', such as eCoaches can be designed. Such digitisation of health-related risks enables the enrolment of individuals into programmes that encourage taking responsibility for their own health, whereby these risks can be controlled by professionals, political bodies or other actors. This intervention in individuals' personal lives shifts to increasingly earlier points in time, challenging individual autonomy and choice.

Given the timeframe of this study (during the development of the eCoaches and strategies), it was neither possible to include users' understandings of and responses to the constructed risks and proposed solutions discussed here nor their potential discursive creation of *other* risks. Because understandings of risk may play out differently as users engage with eCoaches in practice, future research should also examine (discursive) constructions and understandings of digital risk from the perspective of the users of these technologies.

Disclosure statement

No potential conflict of interest was reported by the authors.

Funding

The Socially Robust e-Coaching (SReC) project is funded by the Dutch Partnership Programme 'Healthy Lifestyle Solutions' of STW, NIHC and Philips Research (Project number 13293).

References

Adam, B., & van Loon, J. (2000). Introduction: Repositioning risk; the challenge for social theory. In B. Adam, U. Beck, & J. van Loon (Eds.), *The Risk Society and Beyond. Critical Issues for Social Theory* (pp. 1–31). London: Sage.

Adams, S. A., & De Bont, A. A. (2007). Information Rx: Prescribing good consumerism and responsible citizenship. *Health Care Analysis, 15*(4), 273–290. doi:10.1007/s10728-007-0061-9

Beck, G., & Kropp, C. (2011). Infrastructures of risk: A mapping approach towards controversies on risks. *Journal of Risk Research, 14*(1), 1–16. doi:10.1080/13669877.2010.505348

Beck, U. (1992). *Risk society. Towards a new modernity.* London: Sage.

Beck-Gersheim, E. (2000). Health and responsibility: From social change to technological change and vice versa. In B. Adam, U. Beck, & J. van Loon (Eds.), *The Risk Society and Beyond. Critical Issues for Social Theory* (pp. 122–135). London: Sage.

Bernard, H. R. (1994). *Research methods in anthropology: Qualitative and quantitative approaches* (2nd ed.). London: Sage.

Boenink, M., Swierstra, T., & Stemerding, D. (2010). Anticipating the Interaction between Technology and Morality: A Scenario Study of Experimenting with Humans in Bionanotechnology. *Studies in Ethics, Law, and Technology, 4*(2). doi:10.2202/1941-6008.1098

Brown, R. C. H. (2013). Moral responsibility for (un)healthy behaviour. *Public Health Ethics, 39*, 695–698.

Crawford, R. (2006). Health as meaningful social practice. *Health: An Interdisciplinary Journal for the Social Study of Health, Illness and Medicine, 10*(4), 401–420.

Creswell, J. W. (1998). *Qualitative inquiry and research design: Choosing among five designs.* London: Sage.

Dean, H. (2000). Managing risk by controlling behaviour: Social security administration and the erosion of welfare citizenship. In P. Taylor-Gooby (Ed.), *Risk, trust and welfare* (pp. 51–70). Basingstoke, UK: St. Martin's Press.

Dickenson, D. (2013). *Me medicine vs. we medicine: Reclaiming biotechnology for the common good.* New York, NY: Columbia University Press.

Douglas, M. (1990). Risk as a forensic resource. *Daedalus, 119*(4), 1–16.

Douglas, M., & Wildavsky, A. (1983). *Risk and culture: An essay on the selection of technological and environmental dangers.* Berkeley, CA: University of California Press.

Felt, U., Bister, M. D., Strassnig, M., & Wagner, U. (2009). Refusing the information paradigm: Informed consent, medical research and patient participation. *Health, 13*(1), 87–106.

Fogg, B. J. (2002). *Persuasive technology: Using computers to change what we think and do*. San Francisco, CA: Morgan Kaufmann Publishers.

Foucault, M. (1991). 'Governmentality', trans. Rosi Braidotti and revised by Colin Gordon. In G. Burchell, C. Gordon, & P. Miller (Eds.), *The foucault effect: Studies in governmentality* (pp. 87–104). Chicago, IL: University of Chicago Press.

Green, J., & Thorogood, N. (2004). *Qualitative methods for health research*. London: Sage.

Harris, R., Wyatt, S., & Wathen, N. (Eds.). (2010). *Configuring health consumers: Health work and the imperative of personal responsibility*. Houndmills, UK: Palgrave.

Hooker, C., Carter, S. M., & Davey, H. (2009). Writing the risk of cancer: Cancer risk in public policy. *Health, Risk & Society*, *11*(6), 541–560. doi:10.1080/13698570903329458

Krueger, R. A., & Casey, M. A. (2000). *Focus Groups* (3rd ed.). London: Sage.

Lucivero, F. (2013). The promises of emerging diagnostics: From scientists' visions to the lab bench and back. In S. Burg & T. Swierstra (Eds.), *Ethics on the laboratory floor: Towards a cooperative ethics for the development of responsible technology* (pp. 151–167). Houndmills, UK: Palgrave.

Lupton, D. (1993). Risk as moral danger: The social and political functions of risk discourse in public health. *International Journal of Health Services*, *23*(3), 425–435. doi:10.2190/16AY-E2GC-DFLD-51X2

Lupton, D. (1999). *Risk*. London: Routledge.

Lupton, D. (2006a). Risk and governmentality. In J. F. Cosgrave (Eds.), *The sociology of risk and gambling reader* (pp. 85–99). New York, NY: Taylor & Francis.

Lupton, D. (2006b). Sociology and risk. In G. Mythen & S. Walklate (Eds.), *Beyond the risk society: Critical reflections on risk and human security* (pp. 11–24). Maidenhead: McGraw-Hill Education.

Lupton, D. (2012). M-Health and health promotion: The digital cyborg and surveillance society. *Social Theory & Health*, *10*(3), 229–244. doi:10.1057/sth.2012.6

Lupton, D. (2013). *Digitized health promotion: Personal responsibility for health in the web 2.0 era* (Working paper). Retrieved from http://ses.library.usyd.edu.au/bitstream/2123/9190/1/Working%20paper%20No.%205%20-%20Digitized%20health%20promotion.pdf

Lupton, D. (2015). Health promotion in the digital era: A critical commentary. *Health Promotion International*, *30*(1), 174–183. doi:10.1093/heapro/dau091

Rose, N., O'Malley, P., & Valverde, M. (2006). Governmentality. *Annual Reviews Law Social Sciences*, *2*, 83–104. doi:10.1146/annurev.lawsocsci.2.081805.105900

Singleton, V. (2005). The Promise of Public Health: Vulnerable Policy and Lazy Citizens. *Society and Space*, *23*(5), 771–786. doi:10.1068/d355t

Strauss, A. L., & Corbin, J. M. (1990). *Basics of qualitative research: Grounded theory procedures and techniques*. London: Sage.

STW Website. (2011). Healthy lifestyle solutions programme description (in Dutch). http://www.stw.nl/nl/content/stw-nihc-en-philips-research-starten-onderzoek-naar-e-coaching-voor-een-gezonder-leven

Swierstra, T., Stemerding, D., & Boenink, M. (2009). Exploring techno-moral change: The case of the obesity pill. In P. Sollie & M. Düwell (Eds.), *Evaluating new technologies* (Vol. 3, pp. 119–138). Dordrecht: Springer.

Taylor-Gooby, P. (2008). Sociological approaches to risk: Strong in analysis but weak in policy influence in recent UK developments. *Journal of Risk Research*, *11*(7), 863–876. doi:10.1080/13669870701876592

Van Asselt, M., & Renn, O. (2011). Risk governance. *Journal of Risk Research*, *14*(4), 431–449. doi:10.1080/13669877.2011.553730

Digitalised health, risk and motherhood: politics of infant feeding in post-colonial Hong Kong

Sau Wa Mak

Department of Anthropology, The Chinese University of Hong Kong, Shatin, New Territories, Hong Kong

In 2013, the 'right to baby formula' movement supported by educated, middle-class Chinese families in Hong Kong was launched online challenging the dominant message that 'breast is best'. In this article, I focus on links between mediatisation, globalisation of formula milk and motherhood in post-colonial Hong Kong. Although previous research has examined ideologies of motherhood and mothers' infant feeding decisions, little research has focused on the impact of digital media within post-colonial societies undergoing rapid social change. Drawing on data from a study of mothers living in Hong Kong that I conducted during 2010–2011 and 2013–2014, I show how digital media contribute to changes in individuals' experiences with breastfeeding, perceptions of risk and health, as well as social relations, norms, values and identities in contemporary Hong Kong. I explore how and with what consequences the family, especially as it relates to motherhood and childhood, and the practices of infant feeding are intertwined with digital media and the body politic in neoliberal, post-colonial Hong Kong. I argue that although digital media have globalised the biomedical discourse that 'breast is best', mothers in Hong Kong have, through digital storytelling and virtual interaction, generated alternative interpretations of science, health and their embodied illness experience that serve to counterbalance the cultural contradictions of motherhood. I show that through social networking, parents have not only gained sufficient political power to secure formula milk, they are also simultaneously subsumed to consumer desire created by the marketing of international pharmaceutical companies.

Introduction

In 2013, a group of educated, middle-class Hong Kong citizens became so agitated by potential health risks posed by formula milk shortages that they submitted the petition 'Baby Hunger Outbreak in Hong Kong, International Aid Requested' on the White House website, asking the United States to intervene on their behalf (Tsang, Chiu, & Nip, 2013).

Local parents in Hong Kong can hardly buy baby formula milk powder in drugstores and supermarkets, as smugglers from mainland China have stormed into this tiny city to buy milk powder and resell it for huge profits in China. ... We request international support and assistance, as babies in Hong Kong will face malnutrition very soon. (White House, United States government, 2013)

Within a few days, 13,400 individuals have signed the petition (Chen, 2013) making this 'Baby Hunger Outbreak' petition one of a series of civil movements created by Hong Kong parents to secure their babies' consumption of formula milk. These parents claimed that the shortage of formula milk was a great health risk to infants and young children in Hong Kong, where the breastfeeding rate after the first month is only 2.3%. Such events in this 'right to baby formula' movement seem to contradict trends in many western societies, where the mainstream medical discourse is that 'breast is best' and formula-feeding is believed to increase health risks to babies and mothers.

In this article, I examine how digital media have reconfigured perceptions of health, the framing and communication of risk, infant feeding choices and the performance of motherhood. I focus my analysis on Hong Kong, a rapidly changing post-colonial, post-industrial society.

Mothering in a digitalised, post-colonial risk society

Perceiving oneself as at-risk is the way of being and ruling in the world of modernity (Beck, 2006). The climate of risk is fundamental to the way that both lay people and experts in contemporary societies organise the social world (Giddens, 1991, p. 123). Risk communication, assessment and management dominate a wide range of current political programmes and professional practices, not least in the health field. Neoliberal subjects are expected to exercise prudence in the face of such expert risk assessments and to organise and justify their behaviour as responsible and rational responses to actuarial data (Murphy, 2000). Recent studies have demonstrated that social media now play a significant role in the communication of health information, for example of those who use social networking sites, 35% have obtained health information on the site, while 26% have monitored their friends' personal health experiences (Fox, 2013). Web 2.0 has further changed the way that individuals access health information: 34% of Internet users have read someone else's commentary or experience about health or medical issues, and 6% of Internet users have posted comments, questions or information about health or medical issues (Fox, 2011).

A major strand of current literature on mothering and infant feeding in risk societies focuses on the ideology of intensive mothering and its influence on women's decisions on whether to breastfeed. Successful child-rearing is defined as 'child-centred' (Lee, 2008) and risk-averse (Furedi, 2002). 'Good mothers' are 'risk managers', solely responsible for meeting their children's needs and for taking measures to minimise potential risks posed to their children by food and feeding-related consumer items (Afflerback, Carter, Anthony, & Grauerholz, 2013, Avishai, 2007; Furedi, 2002; Hays, 1996; Lee, 2007, 2008; Murphy, 1999; Stearns, 2009). One prominent, explicit version of intensive mothering is the attachment parenting philosophy (Eyer, 1992; Kukla, 2005), which requires physical closeness – facilitated by breastfeeding, baby-wearing and co-sleeping – said to promote bonding and facilitate immediate maternal responsiveness to the baby's cues. The recent resurgence in popularity of breastfeeding can reasonably be explained by this ideology of 'intensive mothering'. In addition, breast milk is considered superior to formula because breastfeeding provides protection from many diseases and reduces health risks for both mother and child (Carter, Reyes-Foster, & Rogers, 2015). Breastfeeding mothers in contemporary western societies have come to be respected as 'good mothers' (Ludlow et al., 2012), while those who formula-feed are labelled 'bad mothers'.

However, this resurgence has not occurred in Hong Kong, which has one of the lowest rates of breastfeeding in the developed world (Callen & Pinelli, 2004; Chan, Nelson,

Leung, & Li, 2000, Foo, Quek, Ng, Lim, & Deurenberg-Yap, 2005). In 2012, only 2.3% of babies in Hong Kong were being breastfed at the age of 6 months, one of the lowest among regions or countries worldwide (LKS Faculty of Medicine, Hong Kong University, 2014). Furthermore, while in most high-income countries where the breastfeeding rate tend to decline along with family income and education level (Thulier & Mercer, 2009; Wright, Parkinson, & Scott, 2006), in Hong Kong, there is U-curve, with breastfeeding rates among middle-class mothers in Hong Kong being lower than the rates for mothers with upper and lower social class backgrounds (Tarrant et al., 2010). There has been little systematic research into the factors which shape women's choices on infant feeding. Alaszewski, in his analysis of everyday living with risk, suggests the importance of understanding risk framing and communications in affecting human behaviour (Alaszewski, 2005; Alaszewski & Coxon, 2008). One possible approach for understanding the popularity of bottle-feeding in Hong Kong, among the middle-class mothers in particular, is to study how they frame various risks associated with infant feeding and their effects on mothers' social and cultural identities. Risk is socially and culturally mediated, and risk framing is related to personal biography with a social and moral dimension (Alaszewski 2006; Lupton, 2003; Tulloch, 2008). Alaszewski points out that risk consciousness and associated decision-making are often related more to the emotive consequences and meanings attached to certain identified risks than to any rational calculation of probability (Alaszewski, 2005; see also Kasperson & Kasperson, 1996, 2005). Dabrowska and Wismer (2010), in their study of Old Order Mennonites in Ontario, Canada, note that mothers' perceptions of children's health are affected by other factors like their adaptability to environmental changes and their resilience to risks.

Researchers have found that the mass media play an important role in risk framing and communications (see for example Gerbner & Gross, 1976). Digital media are a recent development of the mass media and included information and communications encoded in machine-readable formats and include social media, websites, digital imagery and video, MP3s and e-books. Digital media and networks have become embedded in everyday life in high-income countries and have become part of the broad-based changes in the ways in which individuals in those societies engage in knowledge production, communication and creative expression (Bennett, 2008). Livingstone and Ranjana (2010) found that interactive and mobile technologies are contributing to important changes in family relations and practices in contemporary western societies. However, to date there has been little systematic study of the ways in which digital media affect health risk perceptions, maternal identity and infant feeding in rapidly changing post-colonial societies.

In this article, I aim to develop the understanding of infant feeding and maternal identity in highly developed countries, by studying infant feeding in Hong Kong and considering the ways in which the historical and political context of this post-colonial city influences infant feeding practices. Some of the major social and political changes affecting mothers' livelihoods since the transfer of power in 1997 from the UK to the People's Republic of China include the change in the language of instruction in schools, the privatisation of education and the emergence of resource competition with new migrants from mainland China.

One of the most important changes in educational policy in post-colonial Hong Kong has been the change in the language of instruction from English to Chinese. Under British colonial rule, English was used as the medium of instruction in secondary schools. Students were required by their primary or secondary schools to choose an English personal name and most continued to use their self-chosen English personal names alongside there given personal Chinese names throughout their lives. Two months after the handover, a new diktat was announced: at the start of the 1998 school year, the medium of instruction in Secondary Forms 1–3 was changed from English to Chinese and only a hundred qualified schools were allowed to retain English. School principals, parents and the students themselves, all criticised the change and there were press conferences, on-street protests and letters of appeal to newspapers (see for example *Ming Pao*, 4 December 1997). English has been a form of social and cultural capital for Hong Kong people since the start of the twentieth century. Being proficient in English ensured that an individual enjoyed political and social privileges during the colonial era, and has continued to bestow an economic advantage following Hong Kong's development into a global centre of commerce (Chan, 2002). Since reunification, Hong Kong has strived to maintain its leading international role position despite rapid growth among Chinese cities on the mainland, so much so that the assertion of its international status has become the *raison d'être* of the city-state (Chan, 2002, Chen, 2010; Chiu & Lui, 2009). To maintain its claim to being a 'global city', the administration and media in Hong Kong seek to enhance its standing in major international ranking exercise such as the World Economic Forum's 'Global Competitiveness Report'.

As the decline in Hong Kong's regional competitiveness has made regular headlines in the media, Hong Kong people have taken internationalisation ever more seriously, leading to a surge in the demand and supply of 'international' primary schools and kindergartens. This shift began at the same time that the Hong Kong Special Administrative Region (SAR) government announced its aspiration to develop the city-state into a regional education hub through aggressive development of the higher education sector, despite withholding its commitment to compulsory schooling – such as cutting class sizes – and privatising primary and secondary schools (Choi, 2005, Education Commission, 2000, p. 146). Although the administration has imposed Chinese as the medium of instruction in state schools, it has created a direct subsidy system in which a small number of schools (Education and Manpower Bureau 2004a) receive a government subsidy based on a per-capita rate but are free to choose the medium of instruction, curriculum, school fees and entrance requirements (Education and Manpower Bureau 2004b). The rationale behind these initiatives is to nurture the city's 'brainpower', and this coupled with the city's status as a global financial centre is designed to ensure Hong Kong has the capacity to attracting and retaining the best talent. This 'soft power' is designed to protect the city's status as a regional hub (Cheung, 2009).

In addition to the change in the language of school instruction and the decline in Hong Kong's economic competitiveness, another source of growing anxiety and insecurity among Hong Kong people has been increasing competition for resources, especially education resources, with migrants from China. The media coined the term 'The Great Kindergarten Scare' to refer to Hong Kong parents' anxiety over the level of competition to gain a spot in a local kindergarten for the 2014 school year. This scare has been attributed to the thousands of mainland parents of children born in Hong Kong who applied for kindergarten places for the 2014 school year, and local parents have queued at several kindergartens to obtain the coveted slots. It was reported in media at that time that at some preschools with easy accessibility or particularly good reputations, roughly four out of every five parents in the queues came from the mainland (Chan & Kao, 2013).

Given the special history of Hong Kong and its distinctive social and economic situation, in this article, I explore a number of themes. I start by considering how middle-class mothers in Hong Kong frame the health risks associated with infant feeding. I consider the kind of risks these mothers identify in their attempts to adjust to the rapid sociopolitical changes in post-colonial Hong Kong and how might those changes affect mothers' perceptions of risks posed to health and to their cultural identities. I explore the role the media play in risk framing, risk communication, health knowledge construction and bodily experience among the middle-class mothers who, as discussed, have a lower breastfeeding rate, compared with the upper and lower social classes. I examine Chinese women's narratives about breastfeeding and their experiences with formula-hunting provide insights in the context of mediatisation (the process by which contemporary society has become dependent on the media and its logic (Asp, 1990; Hjarvard, 2009)), social policy and the body.

Methodology

Design

In this article, I use a case-study approach to explore how digital media affect the circulation of medical and health information, and how digital media shape the Chinese mothers' bodily experiences, as well as frame and communicate the risks associated with their choice of infant feeding practices in post-colonial Hong Kong.

To understand the individual experiences of middle-class mothers in Hong Kong in formula-feeding or breastfeeding their infants and young children, mothers' process of rationalisation for their decisions on infant feeding and their understanding of their duties as mothers, amidst the increasing publicity surrounding breast milk as the best food for babies, I used multiple case studies approach with data collected from a variety of sources, including in-depth interviews, popular parenting websites, personal blogs and the Facebook profiles of the mothers so as to give a full picture of this cultural phenomenon (Baxter & Jack, 2008).

Data collection and analysis

In this study, I recruited the informants of my case studies by snowball sampling method through my social network. As Bott has noted, social networks provide a way of recruiting of informants for sensitive topics, such as conjugal relationships and self-identity (Bott, 1971). I restricted the sample size for case studies to 20 so that I could get to know individuals and families as intimately as possible, given my own position as a breastfeeding, middle-class, educated Chinese mother with a young son (I told the participants in my study about my feeding choices, my work as a social researcher and my mother/wife status). I start the snowballing process from my immediate social network, my school and university peers and relatives. The majority of individuals in my social network were middle class, in terms of their occupations, level of education (at least higher education) and ability to speak English. They were middle class in the sense that they were neither wealthy nor poor (see Forrest, La Grange, & Ngai-ming, 2002). The median age of interview participants was 35, although the women ranged in age from 24 to 65. All the 20 women I interviewed used digital media intensively. They connected with friends, colleagues and family members on Facebook and by webchat, and all of them used Web-connected smartphones. Half checked their online email or Facebook accounts approximately hourly on weekdays and most searched daily for parenting and other information online. I was aware that snowball sampling can result in wrong anchoring in an atypical group and community bias (Morgan, 2008). I attempted to overcome these limitations by beginning with an initial set of participants that were as diverse as possible, including individuals working in the insurance, banking, architecture, advertising and accounting industries, as well as a few individuals working in medical or health-related fields as doctors, nutritionists and nurses.

In this article, I draw on data from multiple case studies conducted in Hong Kong for my doctoral research between 2011 and 2012 plus additional research in 2014 and 2015. During my initial year-long fieldwork, I conducted in-depth interviews using a semi-structured, open-ended interview guide with couples who had at least one child aged 3 years or younger. These interviews were separated into two parts – one session each for the mothers and fathers – with each session lasting between 1 and 2 hours. In the process of data collection, I followed the ethical guideline set by the Association of Social Anthropology. I use pseudonyms for participants in this article. The original study encompassed a range of prenatal and postnatal experience, dietary changes, health beliefs and gender relationships in the family and work. However, in my conversations with mothers about their knowledge, experience and decision-making processes on infant feeding, digital media emerged as a key part of the motherhood experience and a key source of information about infant feeding. In this article, I focus on and use the data from the interview components related to digital media, mothers' thoughts, decisions and experiences with infant feeding.

To encompass new developments taking place between 2014 and 2015, I conducted follow-up interviews with the same 20 mothers using a guided conversation approach. I talked to each participant for an hour to an hour and a half. These conversations usually took place in informal social settings such as the participant's home, or in restaurants and playgrounds and moved freely over a range of domestic topics such as family matters and baby feeding. The participants generally did not want their conversations audio-recorded so I took notes during the conversation which I wrote up as soon as possible afterwards.

I subjected the interview data to detailed inductive analysis and developed a coding framework on the basis of five chosen cases. I specified operational definitions of codes and incorporated then in a coding handbook which I amended as I refined the codes. I then applied the revised framework to all of the interview transcripts.

With my informants' consent, I also accessed and studied their blogs and Facebook pages, as well as the most popular parenting website in Hong Kong, Baby-Kingdom.com, for the periods from 2011 to 2012 and 2014 to 2015 to discern mothers' views on infant feeding. Since bottle-feeding is the norm in Hong Kong, most of the women I interviewed had no hesitation in telling me about the problems they had encountered in their attempts at breastfeeding and the process of switching to infant formula or to mixing breastfeeding with formula-feeding. To understand these decisions, I will explore some of these women's narratives on their infant feeding decisions.

Findings

Tiffany, the mother of a 6-month-old baby, posted the following comment on www.Baby-Kingdom.com (the largest Chinese-language parenting website in Hong Kong with 333,000 members from 100,000 families, in 2015 the site had 780,000 visitors a month who viewed over 30 million pages) expressing her frustration in trying to obtain a can of the most popular imported formula milk brand:

> Thanks to the big customers from China, all of Mead Johnson's Stage One formula milk for babies under six months old is 20% more expensive than usual. Even if you can pay the price, it is all out of stock! Hong Kong babies need to feed on shit! Will the Hong Kong government

only intervene when our babies are dying? (Tiffany, Baby-Kingdom.com 2011, original posted in Chinese)

Tiffany viewed formula milk as essential for the well-being of her baby and other babies in Hong Kong. Her concern that wealthy shoppers from mainland China posed a threat to the life chances and well-being of her baby was hardly unique. I found that such anxieties were shared by the majority of the participants in my study.

Digitalised work and the risk of lack-of-milk syndrome

All of the 20 mothers I interviewed had tried to breastfeed their babies, but only, Susan Yeung, was still breastfeeding 6 months after the birth of her baby. All of the other mothers had rapidly switched from breastfeeding to formula-feeding within 2 months of the birth of their babies.

   Alice Kwan, a 46-year-old insurance manager at an international insurance company who switched to formula milk in the second week after giving birth to her third daughter, talked about the ways in which the pressure of her job shaped her decision in the following way:

> When I returned from the hospital, some of my clients called me and I had to follow up on their insurance orders. These were urgent matters, as they needed to claim their money. I had to help them even though I was on maternity leave. Nowadays, if you don't respond quickly, you are out. If your clients can do everything by themselves online, they don't need you. In the first week after delivery, when I put my baby to my breast, she sucked and sucked, and then started to cry. I tried to pump the milk out, but I could hardly squeeze out 2 ounces of milk. I didn't breast feed my two elder daughters, who are now 22 and 17, at all. Nobody talked about the benefits of breast feeding in the 1980s and 1990s, you know. Nowadays, we all know that breast feeding is good.

In her account she blamed her body, it was incapable of producing enough milk. In her conversation she described how she had tried to be a good mother by buying the latest technology to support her breastfeeding but had that when she had doubt about her body, she had used the social media as a source of advice:

> Some of my friends had shared their experiences with breast feeding on their Facebook profiles, and I was very determined to try breast feeding my third baby. I spent over a thousand dollars on buying all the equipment necessary for supplying breast milk – an electronic breast pump, sterilised plastic milk sacks, the bra for nursing, breast pads – but I found myself unsure whether I had sufficient milk for my baby. I asked myself, *Should I continue to breast feed?* I didn't want to share this with my husband or relatives. Talking to them always just makes me more confused. So, I went to Baby-Kingdom.com to ask for advice. I felt so relieved to receive an immediate response from another mum in the middle of the night. She had also faced a similar problem before. She told me that 2 oz. of milk per feeding was not sufficient for a seven-day old baby. What she had done was to mix this with formula milk. I decided to follow her example and started combining breast feeding with formula-feeding. It worked!

The women I talked to tended not to judge the success of their efforts to breastfeed in terms of the reactions and health condition of the baby, such as observed weight gain, but instead focused on quantity of milk that they were able to pump out from their bodies. This approach was facilitated by new equipment for breastfeeding – in this case, the breast milk pump. This technology has only became available on the market in the last two decades and only become common in Hong Kong in the past decade years and is now widely discussed in digital media on popular parenting websites such as Baby-Kingdom. com and MammyDaddy.com and on women's personal blogs and on Facebook. Such media provide mothers such as Alice with new social spaces to meet and chat virtually with other mothers, as well as providing resources for alternative interpretations of medical science and an understanding of 'insufficient milk' as being expressed by the quantity of milk, which deviates from formal medical discourse.

Nicole Lai is a 32-year-old senior journalist at one of the top-selling print media agencies in Hong Kong. Like Alice, her working conditions have changed dramatically due to the growth in popularity of the Internet. Nicole described her strategy of decreasing her workload before giving birth in an attempt to improve the health of her unborn foetus, as well as to improve her baby's health after birth through breastfeeding:

> Once I learned I was pregnant, I decided I would breast feed. I had read a lot about the benefits of breast feeding, such as better nutrition. One key factor in successful breast feeding, which I learnt from parenting magazines and websites, is that I should not be stressed out, so I decided to change jobs. I used to work in the daily newspaper department, with tight deadlines and long working hours. Our work had also become more intense following the launch of our online news website. Now video and instant news have to be uploaded almost immediately from the news collection. So, I requested to change to the weekly magazine department six months before I was scheduled to give birth.

Nicole started breastfeeding but 2 weeks after giving birth she shifted to formula-feeding. Like Alice, she blamed her body for not producing enough describing it as having 'lack-of-milk syndrome'. She described her failure in the following way:

> However, it was a big blow for me when I wasn't able to produce enough milk to feed my daughter. She kept crying after each short suckling in the first few days. I was shocked, depressed and totally unprepared to handle this. I didn't even have a can of formula milk or baby formula at home, you know. *What's wrong with me?*, I thought. Shouldn't every mother be able to breast feed?

Like Alice, Nicole checked for baby feeding information on parenting websites. She felt less of a failure when she learnt that 'lack-of-milk syndrome' was common among her middle-class, same-age peer group, who usually hold senior positions in large organisations and wait to give birth until their mid- to late thirties. She said she was reassured and inspired by a mother's post entitled 'Why successful women cannot breast feed'. The post included an account of a prenatal seminar in which an experienced nurse stated that many career women in Hong Kong were high achievers and perfectionists who pushed themselves so hard that they sometimes even forgot to eat. The nurse said that these women preferred to pump their milk rather than directly feeding it to their baby so that they could measure exactly how much their babies was receiving. However, the nurse noted that this could create stress and inhibit the production of breast milk and as a result many of these educated professional women who pumped milk came to think that they did not have enough milk and stopped breastfeeding.

The 'lack-of-milk syndrome' discourse was widely circulated in social media and also resonated with many of the participants in my study. Rebecca Chan, a 43-year-old senior graphic designer, articulated this 'lack-of-milk syndrome' in the following way blaming the failure of the body on stressful modern life:

I know that breast milk is good for the baby. But it is beyond my control. I formula-feed my son simply because I have no milk. This is what we modern women have to face, isn't it? Long work hours, no exercise and an unhealthy diet. Our lives are too stressful for breast feeding. We are simply too tired.

Thus, Alice, Nicole and Rebecca all explained the 'lack-of-milk syndrome' in terms of the pressure on working middle-class mothers who had to deal with the demands of work and other expectations while feeding their babies. Despite producing 'insufficient milk', many mothers posting on Baby-Kingdom.com expressed varying degrees of guilt and a sense of failure at being unable to breastfeed. From the parenting websites, mothers receive notes of encouragement in the form of success stories on breastfeeding, as well as discussions of modern mothering that stress the social role of giving 'quality time and care' to babies rather than solely emphasising the biological role of breastfeeding. The breastfeeding mothers also share pragmatic information, such as where to buy milk pumps and other equipment, and the dietary guidelines for stimulating breast-milk production.

The development of the digital media not only changes the personal and private life, it was also changing the work environment, as Alice noted. The Internet has transformed business models globally, and these women work in industries that have undergone great changes – such as reorganisations in corporate structure and job nature – in the digital era. Insurance products can now be sold online, threatening the role of insurance agents as intermediaries and meaning that working mothers had to adjust to these new work environment if they were to survive. Yet, the digital media could also facilitate breastfeeding by creating the possibility of flexible working conditions given sympathetic employers. Susan Yeung's account provides an important contrast to the experiences recounted above. As a senior journalist specialising in Hong Kong and China financial politics, with a regular personal column in a local English newspaper, she described how her employers had enabled her to work flexibly and this had enabled her to deal with the challenges of breastfeeding:

Breast feeding is difficult for modern women! No one told me that breast feeding is so tiring. ... I breast fed my daughter almost ten times a day in the first three weeks and I always felt nervous about whether I could produce sufficient milk. Luckily, my editor has allowed me to cut my workload. Now, I only go to the office for one day and work at home for the rest of the week.

As a well-established columnist, Susan felt she had the social, cultural and economic capital to bargain for greater flexibility in her working time and place. Her employer trusted her and was willing to let her work flexibly. She described how she used the Internet to access to international news, media and her company's online database and in her case, the digital media enabled her to work from home and continue breastfeeding her child. Like the other participants in my study, Susan visited and made use of digital media such as the Baby Kingdom site, for tips about breastfeeding but she said she preferred to use her own social network to discuss intimate issues about child care:

I visit Baby Kingdom regularly and I have received a lot of good breast feeding tips, such as where to buy a milk pump. However, I am not the kind of person who can share my stories with strangers. I feel more comfortable talking to my mummy friends and seeking 'real' childcare support from my family, especially my sister. After the first month, everything seemed on track – we were both eating and sleeping well. My daughter is now turning two and I am still breast feeding. She is a happy, healthy girl. I feel that I have done the best thing for her by breast feeding.

In her conversations, Susan attributed her success in breastfeeding in part to following 'traditional' advice such as using her mother's recipe to make 'blood-enhancing' Chinese soups:

> To ensure that I can produce sufficient milk, I drink a lot of fish soup based on my mother's recipe and I eat a big sandwich before bed, as suggested by my mid-wife when I gave birth in the United Kingdom.

The participants in my study attributed the 'lack-of-milk syndrome' to an imbalance in the body's state caused by the stress of working in a digitalised environment. They described the ways in which traditional Chinese foods could be used to counter this imbalance and family members and friends shared traditional soup recipes (including fish and papaya soup, ginger and vinegar soup and heidou cha (black bean tea soup) for enhancing breast milk production and these recipes were widely circulated via the Internet.

Digitalised risk, intensive mothering and the education imperative

Winnie Cheung, a 31-year-old merchandising manager in a garment factory, told me how she started using formula milk a month after her baby was born due to feelings of fatigue, though this fatigue was not so much due to work as to the demands of the educational system:

> When my son was three months old, my neighbours kept asking me which playgroup he would be attending. I told them that I hadn't signed up for any and they looked at me like I had done something wrong. I felt nervous and began scouring online parenting and education forums for the most popular school choices. I felt even more stressed when I learnt how intense the competition in the good, child-oriented primary schools is. Our kids are not only competing with kids from Hong Kong but also those from China. I have read newspaper articles saying that wealthy mainlanders are buying houses in Kowloon Tong to ensure that their only sons have a higher chance of entering one of the elite primary schools in the area.

Many of participants in my study told me that they had similar anxieties and felt great fatigue – as if they were preparing for an epic battle – when faced with enrolling their children in kindergarten. Peggy Ho, a 39-year-old entrepreneur, shared the importance of her child's schooling for her child and for her family, and reflected on how this might affect mothers' decisions on breastfeeding:

> I think the most important thing for a mother nowadays is to make sure that your son or daughter can enter into a good school – an English-speaking one with students from other parts of the world, like Europe and America. This is almost the *only* thing that parents and even grandparents talk about in workplaces, at friends' gatherings, in tea houses and on Facebook. I learnt from Facebook that almost all my university classmates' children were admitted into reputable schools. I will feel ashamed if my son can't get into one.

Peggy explained to me how the health information via digital media affected her decisions regarding infant feeding:

> I learnt from the breast feeding mothers on the parenting websites that they need to feed the babies ten times a day! I think this is too much for me. ... To be honest, nobody cares whether you breast feed or not, so long as your son gets into a good school. I have met so many parents and even grandparents who introduce their kids and grandchildren in terms of the names of the schools they attend instead of by their individual names. We will be labelled

as 'bad' mothers if our children cannot get into these elite schools. Like the mother of Mengzi [an exemplary Chinese historical role model who is reported to have moved the family home three times so her son could be near a school that fostered his scholarly development], we Hong Kong mothers torture ourselves to ensure our children's educational opportunities and to ensure a better life for them. I think I would rather use my time and energy to prepare for my son's schooling than to bother about breast feeding.

Thus Peggy, like most of the participants in my study, was more concerned about the risk that her baby would not get the 'right' education rather than the risk she would not right type of feed. Most of the participants in my study told me that before their baby was 6 months old they had attended at least three preschool information sessions or open days and by the time their child was 2 years old they had sent more than eight preschool application forms. Mothers in my study described how getting one's children into a 'good' English-speaking kindergarten was the most important maternal responsibility. Winnie's and Peggy's narratives show being a 'good mother' in Hong Kong was defined not so much by one's choice of infant feeding practice as by which schools one's children enter. Most of the mothers in my study described how formula-feeding was a strategy they used to free up time and energy for pursuing their project of gaining admission to elite schools for their children.

Digitalised health information, e-marketing and online prestige

Amy Cheung, a 26-year-old executive officer at a university, was among the women who switched to a mixture of breast milk and infant formula 6 weeks after the birth of her baby. She talked about her experience of visiting a manufacturer's website, the Mead Johnson, in the following way:

> Since I didn't have enough milk for my daughter, I asked my friends which formula milk they would recommend. They told me that I could make my own decision by getting free formula milk samples from the top-selling brands. I joined Mead Johnson's Mothers' Club, as it has been the number one brand in Hong Kong for the past twelve years. I also liked the auspicious-sounding brand name 'A+', like getting the top grade for my daughter.

For Amy, her use of the website enabled her to deal with the competing demands of being a good mother who made rational decisions on the provision of quality food, monitored her baby's well-being while being frugal with the household's money. Amy described how the pharmaceutical company website provided her with abundant, helpful health information and parenting tips free-of-charge:

> After delivering a sample pack of formula, Mead Johnson has emailed me every month reminding me of my daughter's development stage and the benchmarks for measuring my daughter's growth. I like these emails because they remind me of my daughter's health and developmental condition, and I have found the information to be very reliable, which has saved me time and money in accessing health information.

Amy proudly told me that she and her daughter had recently participated in one of the parenting activities organised by the Mead Johnson, called 'Small kids, Big performance'. In this campaign, parents could register their children to act the roles of a number of reputable professionals, such as doctors, firemen and pilots, in real settings. The funny and unexpected behaviours of Amy's daughter and the other children in these real-life 'make-believe' sessions were recorded on video and uploaded by registered members onto their Facebook profiles, as well as circulated among their friends so as to gain recognition and respect. Amy declared that receiving 103 'Likes' for her daughter's campaign photos on her Facebook profile was one of the greatest accomplishments of her daughter's life.

Charlotte Woo, a 32-year-old computer programme analyst who switched to infant formula 4 weeks after the birth of her baby, described the ways in which her concerns about her son's ability to pass the 'entrance' interview to preschool encouraged her to use the website of another popular formula milk brand, Abbott:

> I am worried about the kindergarten interviews for my son. He is a bit slow in speaking and not quite able to follow instructions. I was attracted by the advertisement of Abbott on their EyeQPlus Classroom. I went to their website, which led me to a series of the most common kindergarten interview questions for children under three years old. After completion, they emailed me a practice certificate, which might be helpful for my son to enter the kindergarten. However, my son couldn't answer most of the questions. I think he needs to catch up in his mental development.

As Charlotte and Amy's narratives show mothers used the corporate websites of pharmaceutical companies for different reasons, ranging from obtaining free formula milk samples to joining child-friendly games or seeking help with kindergarten interview questions. For Amy, Charlotte and like-minded mothers in post-colonial Hong Kong, the digital media provided sites where they could identify the social rules and norms, where they could display their cultural and economic capital and where they were able to sculpt their idealised identities as mothers and as modern women to gain the respect and recognition of their peers. Their use of formula manufacturers' websites, as with many of the other women I interviewed, is not simply an attempt to ensure the basic health and growth of their children, but more about fulfilling their aspirations for mothering – raising smart kids and entering them into the right preschools.

Discussion

In this article, I have analysed some Hong Kong mothers' narratives on their use of digital media, their interpretation of risks and their decisions to formula-feed their babies, against the political context of increasing interaction, reliance on and conflicts with people from China. Mothers' perceptions of their 'lack-of-milk syndrome' and of the associated health and social risks to their babies intersect with their relationships with family members, colleagues and clients in work, as well as with their self-presentation in both the real and the virtual worlds. Such narratives engage reflexively with the social and normative context in which they occur. An analysis of the social function of these accounts is one way in which to illuminate the context of how feeding work is carried out (Murphy, 2000).

To return to the valuable insights offered by Alaszewski (2005) on risk framing, my study also supports a relationship between risk framing and the adaptability of people in a changing environment that may threaten their social and cultural identities. Here, the perception of risk in work and health is affected by the rapid sociopolitical changes in post-colonial Hong Kong and by mothers' personal confidence at coping with these changes. Digital media have dramatically altered the working environment of the middle-class mothers in Hong Kong. Most of my informants work in industries that have undergone great transformations in production, market offerings and promotion methods in the digital era. Insurance products can now be bought and sold online, and daily newspapers now operate like 24-hour TV stations. Staying competitive requires these women to keep connected at all times.

In addition, my findings support the notion that risk framing is related to personal biography, with a social and moral dimension. The societal emphasis on internationalisation and brainpower has been internalised by these mothers as an aspiration to raise their young children as global citizens, with failure to gain entry into a good, English-speaking 'international' preschool perceived not only as affecting the well-being of the young child but also as bringing disgrace to the family.

I found that the digital marketing of the pharmaceutical companies, such as the weekly email on mental and physical health, online learning tools and children's educational events, promoted the idea that intellectual potential and even the future careers of young children was malleable through parental intervention. This finding supports Lupton's suggestion that children's intellectual development is now perceived as an essential part of children's health (Lupton, 2011). Based on her study of mothers in Australia, Lupton contends that it is not only infants' physical health and well-being that is identified in lay accounts as being part of the realm of maternal responsibility. The promotion and stimulation of children's intellectual development has also been incorporated into the list of imperatives to which mothers are expected to respond (Lupton, 2011). As demonstrated by Charlotte's case, for middle-class mothers, potential impacts on a child's intellectual development, both positive and negative, loom large. The child's successful intellectual development has a direct impact on the chances of gaining admission into an English-speaking kindergarten, which was widely believed by my informants to be the first crucial step promoting future success. Having the 'lack-of-milk syndrome', mothers in Hong Kong might see themselves as being a 'risk factor' for their children and to be blamed by the others not only for the current physical condition but also for hindering the intellectual and potential development, and even the social mobility of their children in future.

In my study, I found that the discourse of the 'malleable infant' was promoted mainly through the media and formula milk was marketed as a technology to enhance the intellect, as well as to develop the body, of the infant and young child. This discourse of intellectual enhancement was well received by middle-class mothers, as it accorded with bourgeois ideals of self-improvement, competitiveness and intellectual achievement (Vincent & Ball, 2006). In the face of insecurities in their work and economic potentials, many of my middle-class mothers, who worked long hours in the hopes of advancing their careers, placed their hopes for social mobility on the next generation. These mothers described their use of formula milk as a technology to lower the risks to intellectual development and to increase the competitiveness of their young children in an unforgiving educational market.

On risk communications, my findings support the existence of two-way, interactive communication between knowledgeable experts, which included other women who had already dealt with a situation and occasionally professionals and the uninformed public (Alaszewski, 2005). The mothers in my study were not passive recipients of information; they actively sought out and provided information on the risks associated with education and health. For the women in my study, the digital media tended to intensify their anxieties over potential social risks of the 'kindergarten scare', the health risk of the 'lack-of-milk syndrome' and the feeling of ambiguity among parents, especially mothers, who are raising children in the context of Hong Kong's increasing interaction and reliance upon China.

Digital media have also become a new stage where motherhood is performed and judged. Mothers were concerned about their virtual social status and identity on digital media, such as Facebook, where parenting practices could be compared and contested in more frequent and minute ways. Previous studies on risk and responsibilities associated with mothering in western societies have pointed out that breastfeeding, as promoted by experts, is how a good mother should perform in the risk society under the influence of the powerful ideology of 'intensive mothering'. In Hong Kong, as illustrated by the online rhetoric on the kindergarten scare and formula milk-hunting, the academic competitiveness of young children affects the social status of their mothers and family members. To perform as a good mother, Hong Kong woman prioritise education, creating a norm where ensuring the development of children's capacity for learning is the major health concern. Similar to Hays' description of the intensive mothering practices in America (Hays, 1996), a good middle-class mother in Hong Kong should invest tremendous amounts of time, energy and money in hunting for the right kindergarten.

Not only is digital media a stage in which mothers are able to act the part of good mothers, as demonstrated by my study, but middle-class Chinese mothers increasingly find themselves subject to scrutiny in this new social space. As Lupton had earlier noted, mothers are 'both the subject of surveillance (from other mothers, medical professionals, friends and family members who regularly assess their efforts to promote and protect the health and well-being of their infants) and the instigators of surveillance over their infants and other mothers' (Lupton, 2011). Mothers in Hong Kong were vulnerable to being judged on Facebook and parenting websites on the learning capacity of their children and the ranking of the schools their children have entered, in contrast they were not judged in relationship to their feeding choices. In comparing the high health risk of the 'lack-of-milk syndrome', which may lead to other risks such as intellectual underdevelopment, many Hong Kong mothers choose to devote their time and energy to finding the right schools for their children and to spending quality time with them, rather than breastfeeding. Formula milk can thus be seen as a kind of technology used strategically by Hong Kong mothers to free up their bodies and energy from the duties of lactation, while facilitating their provision of suitable educational opportunities for their children so as to minimise the social and cultural risks they and their children face in future. In this context, the low breastfeeding rate is hardly surprising.

In my study, I also found that trust was important in risk communications (Taylor-Gooby, 2000). The parenting websites provide a new communications channel and social space for mothers to build up friendships with other mothers with similar life courses. Social media, including parenting websites and Facebook, provide a democratic platform on which parents with different life trajectories are able to easily consolidate their personal stories, opinions and energy. Compressing time and space, digital media open up new social spaces for women to share their love and care with one another, to develop trust and to build up self-esteem and gain validation.

At the same time, digital media make alternative interpretations of health, science and bodily experience possible. The 'lack-of-milk syndrome', which aligns with the findings of many quantitative studies conducted on breastfeeding in Hong Kong (Tarrant et al., 2010), is associated with an imbalance in the state of the body caused by work stresses. This bottom-up, non-western health belief is reinforced through social media. Based on traditional Chinese medicine, the 'lack-of-milk syndrome' is the result of a bodily imbalance and can be improved by following special post-partum dietary practices (Furth, 1987).

In a broad sense, the 'lack-of-milk syndrome' represents women's attempts to negotiate the cultural contradictions of motherhood. These modern women are trying to simultaneously embody the social expectations of a successful working woman (professional, hard-working with high income) and of a wise mother who adopts intensive mothering to develop their babies' full potential. The feeling of fatigue, which 'unavoidably' leads to the 'lack-of-milk syndrome', has the moral connotation of a busy career woman who is also a wise, self-sacrificing loving mother that is too exhausted to breastfeed (Lee, 1999). From this perspective, the mothers' perception of having the 'lack-of-milk syndrome' and their feeling of fatigue should not be seen as their real, underlying worries. Rather, the physical experience of the body (breastfeeding, in this case) is always modified by the social categories through which it is known and reflects a particular view of society (Douglas, 1973).

The moral economy of formula-feeding is part and parcel of these mothers' modern identity, an identity which encompasses high social status, economic stability and a modern lifestyle. This modern identity-building process is facilitated by digital media, which allows the creation and dissemination of moral justifications for formula-feeding practices amidst the ubiquity of the ideology of intensive mothering. Formula-feeding is also employed as a technology enabling mothers and their babies to manage future risks related to social immobility, global competition, political change and challenges to Hong Kongers' cultural identity.

Conclusion

In this article, I have highlighted the role that digital media play in framing and communicating health and social risks associated with breastfeeding and other aspect of child-rearing such as schooling, and how this affects the decisions on infant feeding and the cultural identities of middle-class mothers in a post-colonial city. Digital media provide a new channel in which the social risks of children's intellectual development and academic performance are amplified. At the same time, digital media provide a new social space where alternative interpretations of science and health can be exchanged. Mothers can seek love, care and respect from people they trust, and their online words of advice to one another shape mothers' understandings of the 'lack-of-milk syndrome', its associated health risks and the decision on whether to formula-feed, which contests the mainstream health discourse that 'breast is best'. In the process of self-presentation and interaction, new forms, norms and values on health, infant feeding practices and motherhood are created.

Acknowledgements

I thank the women who shared their infant feeding experiences with me. Gratefully, I acknowledge the helpful and thoughtful comments I received from two anonymous reviews. I also thank Prof. Andy Alaszewski for his invaluable help and support, especially in the final stage of revision.

Disclosure statement

No potential conflict of interest was reported by the author.

References

Afflerback, S., Carter, S. K., Anthony, A. K., & Grauerholz, L. (2013). Infant-feeding consumerism in the age of intensive mothering and risk society. *Journal of Consumer Culture, 13*(3), 387–405.

Alaszewski, A. (2005). Risk communication: Identifying the importance of social context. *Health, Risk & Society*, *7*(2), 101–105. doi:10.1080/13698570500148905

Alaszewski, A. (2006). Diaries as a source of suffering narratives: A critical commentary. *Health, Risk & Society*, *8*(1), 43–58. doi:10.1080/13698570500532553

Alaszewski, A., & Coxon, K. (2008). Everyday experience of living with risk and uncertainty. *Health, Risk & Society*, *10*(5), 413–420.

Asp, K. (1990). Medialization, media logic and mediarchy. *Nordicom Review*, *11*(2), 47–50.

Avishai, O. (2007). Managing the lactating body: The breastfeeding project and privileged motherhood. *Qualitative Sociology*, *30*, 135–152. doi:10.1007/s11133-006-9054-5

Baxter, P., & Jack, S. (2008). Qualitative case study methodology: Study design and implementation for novice researchers. *The Qualitative Report*, *13*(4), 544–559.

Beck, U. (2006). Living in the world risk society. *Economy and Society*, *35*(3), 329–345. doi:10.1080/03085140600844902

Bennett, W. L. (2008). Changing citizenship in the digital age. In W. L. Bennett (Ed.), *Civic life online: Learning how digital media can engage youth* (pp. 1–24). The John D. and Catherine T. MacArthur Foundation Series on Digital Media and Learning. Cambridge, MA: The MIT Press.

Bott, E. (1971). *Family and social network: Roles, norms, and external relationships in ordinary urban families*. London: Tavistock Publications.

Callen, J., & Pinelli, J. (2004). Incidence and duration of breastfeeding for term infants in Canada, United States, Europe, and Australia: A literature review. *Birth*, *31*(4), 285–292. doi:10.1111/bir.2004.31.issue-4

Carter, S. K., Reyes-Foster, B., & Rogers, T. L. (2015). Liquid gold or Russian roulette? Risk and human milk sharing in the US news media. *Health, Risk & Society*, *17*(1), 30–45. doi:10.1080/13698575.2014.1000269

Chan, E. (2002). Beyond pedagogy: Language and identity in post-colonial Hong Kong. *British Journal of Sociology of Education*, *23*(2), 271–285. doi:10.1080/01425690220137756

Chan, S., & Kao, E. (2013, October 7). Angry parents protest at mainland Chinese children being given preschool places. *South China Morning Post*.

Chan, S. M., Nelson, E. A. S., Leung, S. S. F., & Li, C. Y. (2000). Breastfeeding failure in a longitudinal post-partum maternal nutrition study in Hong Kong. *Journal of Paediatrics and Child Health*, *36*, 466–471. doi:10.1046/j.1440-1754.2000.00544.x

Chen, P. (2010). *Great cities of the world*. Hong Kong: The University of Hong Kong.

Chen, T. P. (2013). Hong Kong milk formula hotline flooded with calls. *The Wall Street Journal*, China Real Time, 4 February. Retrieved October 25, 2015, from http://blogs.wsj.com/chinarealtime/2013/02/04/hong-kong-milk-formula-hotline-flooded-with-calls/

Cheung, A. B. L. (2009, December 4). *Critical reflections on education change and promoting human capital in Hong Kong*. Paper presented at the Managing Human Capital in World Cities conference, Organised by the Hong Kong Educational Research Association, held in the University of Hong Kong, Hong Kong.

Chiu, S., & Lui, T. L. (Eds.). (2009). *Hong Kong: Becoming a Chinese global city*. London: Routledge.

Choi, P.-K. (2005). A critical evaluation of education reforms in Hong Kong: Counting our losses to economic globalisation. *International Studies in Sociology of Education*, *15*(3), 237–256. doi:10.1080/09620210500200142

Dabrowska, E., & Wismer, S. (2010). Inclusivity matters: Perceptions of children's health and environmental risk including old order Mennonites from Ontario, Canada. *Health, Risk & Society*, *12*(2), 169–188. doi:10.1080/13698571003632445

Douglas, M. (1973). *Natural symbols*. London: The Cresset Press.

Education & Manpower Bureau. (2004a). List of direct subsidy scheme schools 2003/4 and list of schools that will join the direct subsidy scheme in 2004/5. Retrieved November 12, 2015, from http://www.emb.gov.hk/FileManager/EN/Context_175/Schlist2003_e.pdf

Education & Manpower Bureau. (2004b). Getting assessment right – The basic competency assessment. Retrieved November 12, 2015, from http://www.emb.gov.hk/index.aspx?nodeid=2447&langno=1

Education Commission. (2000). *Learning for life, learning through life: Reform proposals for the education system in Hong Kong*. Retrieved November 12, 2015, from http://www.e-c.edu.hk/eng/reform/rfl.html

Eyer, D. (1992). *Mother-infant bonding: A science fiction*. New Haven, CT: Yale University Press.

Foo, L. L., Quek, S. J. S., Ng, S. A., Lim, M. T., & Deurenberg-Yap, M. (2005). Breastfeeding prevalence and practices among Singaporean Chinese, Malay and Indian mothers. *Health Promotion International, 20*(3), 229–237. doi:10.1093/heapro/dai002

Forrest, R., La Grange, A., & Ngai-ming, Y. (2002). Neighbourhood in a high rise, high density city: Some observations on contemporary Hong Kong. *The Sociological Review, 50*(2), 215–240. doi:10.1111/1467-954X.00364

Fox, S. (2011). Peer-to-peer healthcare. *Pew Internet and American Life Project.* Retrieved November 10, 2015, from http://www.pewinternet.org/~/media//Files/Reports/2011/Pew_ P2PHealthcare_2011.pdf

Fox, S. (2013). The social life of health information. *Pew Internet and American Life Project.* Retrieved November 7, 2015, from http://www.pewinternet.org/files/old-media//Files/Reports/ PIP_HealthOnline.pdf

Furedi, F. (2002). *Culture of fear* (revised ed.). London: Continuum.

Furth, C. (1987). Concepts of pregnancy, childbirth and infancy in Ch'ing Dynasty China. *The Journal of Asian Studies, 46*(1), 7–36. doi:10.2307/2056664

Gerbner, G., & Gross, L. (1976). Living with television: The violence profile. *Journal of Communication, 26*(2), 172–194. doi:10.1111/jcom.1976.26.issue-2

Giddens, A. (1991). *Modernity and self-identity.* Cambridge: Polity.

Hays, S. (1996). *The cultural contradictions of motherhood.* New Haven, CT: Yale University Press.

Hjarvard, S. (2009). Soft individualism: Media and the changing social character. In K. Lundby (Ed.), *Mediatization: Concept, changes, consequences* (pp. 159–178). New York, NY: Peter Lang.

Kasperson, J. X., & Kasperson, R. E. (2005). *The social contours of risk.* London: Earthscan.

Kasperson, R. E., & Kasperson, J. X. (1996). The social amplification and attenuation of risk. *The Annals of the American Academy of Political and Social Science, 545*, 95–105. doi:10.1177/ 0002716296545001010

Kukla, R. (2005). *Mass hysteria, medicine, culture and women's bodies.* New York, NY: Roman and Littlefield.

Lee, E. J. (2007). Health, morality, and infant feeding: British mothers' experiences of formula milk use in the early weeks. *Sociology of Health & Illness, 29*(7), 1075–1090. doi:10.1111/j.1467-9566.2007.01020.x

Lee, E. J. (2008). Living with risk in the age of 'intensive motherhood': Maternal identity and infant feeding. *Health, Risk & Society, 10*(5), 467–477. doi:10.1080/13698570802383432

Lee, S. (1999). Fat, fatigue and the feminine: The changing cultural experience of women in Hong Kong. *Culture, Medicine and Psychiatry, 23*(1), 51–73. doi:10.1023/A:1005451614729

Livingstone, S., & Ranjana, D. (2010). Media, communication and information technologies in the European family. *Working Reports: Existential Fields, EF8. Family Platform Project.* Retrieved November 12, 2015, from http://eprints.lse.ac.uk/29788/1/EF8_LSE_MediaFamily_ Education.pdf

LKS Faculty of Medicine, Hong Kong University. (2014). HKU announces a "Children of 1997" cohort study showing breastfeeding's impact on Hong Kong's public health — Baby friendly action joint declaration signed on site to urge for immediate implementation of the HK code. Retrieved November 19, 2015, from http://www.med.hku.hk/v1/news-and-events/press-releases/

Ludlow, V., Newhook, L. A., Newhook, J. T., Bonia, K., Goodridge, J. M., & Twells, L. (2012). How formula feeding mothers balance risks and define themselves as 'good mothers'. *Health, Risk & Society, 14*(3), 291–306. doi:10.1080/13698575.2012.662635

Lupton, D. (2003). *Medicine as culture: Illness, disease and the body.* London: Sage.

Lupton, D. (2011). 'The best thing for the baby': Mothers' concepts and experiences related to promoting their infants' health and development. *Health, Risk & Society, 13*(7–8), 637–651. doi:10.1080/13698575.2011.624179

Morgan, L. D. (2008). *The SAGE encyclopedia of qualitative research methods* (pp. 816–817). Thousand Oaks, CA: SAGE Publications.

Murphy, E. (1999). 'Breast is best': Infant feeding decisions and maternal deviance. *Sociology of Health & Illness, 21*(2), 187–208. doi:10.1111/shil.1999.21.issue-2

Murphy, E. (2000). Risk, responsibility, and rhetoric in infant feeding. *Journal of Contemporary Ethnography, 29*(3), 291–325. doi:10.1177/089124100129023927

Stearns, C. (2009). The work of breastfeeding. *Women Studies Quarterly, 37*(3 & 4), 63–80. doi:10.1353/wsq.0.0184

Tarrant, M., Fong, D. Y., Wu, K. M., Lee, I. L., Wong, E. M., Sham, A., ... Dodgson, J. E. (2010). Breastfeeding and weaning practices among Hong Kong mothers: A prospective study. *BMC Pregnancy and Childbirth*, *10*, 27. doi:10.1186/1471-2393-10-27

Taylor-Gooby, P. (2000). Risk and welfare. In P. Taylor-Gooby (Ed.), *Risk, trust and welfare*. London: Macmillan.

Thulier, D., & Mercer, J. (2009). Variables associated with breastfeeding duration. *Journal of Obstetric, Gynecologic, & Neonatal Nursing*, *38*(3), 259–268. doi:10.1111/jogn.2009.38.issue-3

Tsang, E., Chiu, J., & Nip, A. (2013, January 31). Hongkongers appeal to US over baby formula shortage. *South China Morning Post*.

Tulloch, J. (2008). Risk and subjectivity: Experiencing terror. *Health, Risk & Society*, *10*(5), 451–465. doi:10.1080/13698570802408718

Vincent, C., & Ball, S. (2006). *Childcare, choice and class practices: Middle class parents and their children*. London: Routledge.

White House, United States government. (2013). Retrieved November 18, 2015, from https://petitions.whitehouse.gov/petition/baby-hunger-outbreak-hong-kong-international-aid-requested

Wright, C. M., Parkinson, K., & Scott, J. (2006). Breastfeeding in a UK urban context: Who breastfeeds, for how long and does it matter? *Public Health Nutrition*, *9*(6), 686–691.

'Holy shit, didn't realise my drinking was high risk': an analysis of the way risk is enacted through an online alcohol and drug screening intervention

Michael Savic[a,b], S. Fiona Barker[a,b], Barbara Hunter[a,b] and Dan I. Lubman[a,b]

[a]Turning Point, Eastern Health, Fitzroy, Australia; [b]Eastern Health Clinical School, Faculty of Medicine, Nursing & Health Sciences, Monash University, Box Hill, Australia

Commentators view online screening and automated feedback interventions as low-cost ways of addressing alcohol and other drug-related harms. These interventions place people into categories of risk based upon scores from standardised screens and provide automated feedback about a person's level of risk of developing alcohol and other drug 'problems'. In this article, we examine how one particular alcohol and other drug online screening and feedback intervention enacts risky alcohol and other drug use and users, and explore how these enactments compare to alcohol and other drug users' own accounts of risk. In order to do this, we undertook a qualitative analysis of intervention content and intervention recipients' responses ($n = 489$) to an open-ended question about their experience of the online screening and feedback intervention. Our analysis highlights how the online screening and feedback intervention draws on prevention science to cultivate a sense of expertness and objectivity. Intervention recipients' accounts of risk were either overshadowed by the 'expert' risk account provided by the intervention, 'validated' by the intervention or were not accurately reflected by the intervention. In the latter case, intervention recipient comments draw attention to the way in which the intervention enacts alcohol and other drug use as inherently risky without accounting for the context and purpose of use. While the online screening and feedback intervention assumes that people are capable of self-monitoring and managing their alcohol and other drug use and risk, recommendations for help provided enact intervention recipients as fragile and in need of professional help. We suggest that there is a need for the development of interventions that are better equipped to take account of the complexity of alcohol and other drug use and risk experiences and subjectivities.

Introduction

Public health, psychology and bio-medical discourses have been influential in the characterisation of alcohol and other drug use as inherently risky behaviour that leads to a range of health and social harms (Bunton, 2001; Toumborou, 2002). In response to such characterisations, public health experts and others have developed a number of alcohol and other drug online screening and automated feedback interventions (referred to in this article as online screening and feedback interventions) to manage risk (McCambridge & Cunningham, 2014). While researchers point to the potential for online screening and feedback interventions to reduce alcohol and other drug use or problems (Donoghue, Patton, Phillips, Deluca, & Drummond, 2014; Riper et al., 2014; Sinadinovic, Wennberg, & Berman, 2012), the assumptions behind these interventions, how they enact alcohol and other drug use and users and any unintended consequences, have not been subject to critical analysis. Furthermore, it is not clear how the 'expert' categorisations of risk underpinning online screening and feedback interventions correspond with the accounts of alcohol and other drug use and risk of intervention recipients. Given the tendency for 'expert' accounts of risk to be privileged in drug policy and responses, understanding drug users' own accounts of risk is important in ensuring the appropriateness of interventions and harm reduction responses (Duff, 2003).

In this article, we are not examining the effectiveness of online screening and feedback interventions in reducing alcohol and other drug use or problems. Nor are we questioning the intentions or potential benefits of developing online screening and feedback interventions as ways of engaging people who may not otherwise seek help in discussions about their alcohol and other drug use. Rather we explore how risk, alcohol and other drug use and users are enacted by an online screening and feedback intervention, and how this relates to users' own accounts of risk. Drawing on performative approaches to risk, we view risk in the context of alcohol and other drug use as 'something that is done' (Montelius & Nygren, 2014, p. 433) through practices, objects, discourse and relations rather than something that exists independently of these. In so doing, we argue that the online screening and feedback intervention does not just 'detect' risky alcohol and other drug use and users, but is also implicated in the 'doing', 'enactment' or constitution of risk, alcohol and other drug use and subjectivities.

Screening, feedback interventions and risk

Screening and feedback interventions

Screening and feedback interventions have been viewed as an inexpensive way of addressing alcohol and other drug harms across the population (Babor et al., 2007). They have historically been conducted by health professionals in primary care services, and involve a screening component in which standardised tools, developed by researchers, are used to identify a person's level of risk of experiencing 'real or potential' alcohol and other drug problems (Babor & Higgins-Biddle, 2001, p. 6). Following screening, the health professional typically provides feedback on the person's level of risk and advice about how they could reduce their alcohol and other drug use, as well as offering referral options for people who engage in risky levels of use (Babor et al., 2007). This feedback is thought to 'motivate an individual to do something about' their 'problem' (Babor & Higgins-Biddle, 2001, p. 6), although there is uncertainty about the exact mechanisms through which screening and feedback interventions work (Gaume, McCambridge, Bertholet, & Daeppen, 2014). The entire screening and feedback process can be relatively quick (for example, it can be done in a single session) and requires minimal training to deliver. Given the potential scalability and impact of screening and feedback interventions, they have been increasingly used and evaluated since the late 1980s (McCambridge & Cunningham, 2014).

There has been increased interest in recent years in the online delivery of screening and feedback interventions (McCambridge & Cunningham, 2014). Rather than being delivered by a health professional, online screening and feedback interventions can be self-administered and completed outside of health service settings by an individual gaining direct access to the intervention via the internet (McCambridge & Cunningham, 2014). The user completes the screening test, which uses research-based algorithms to create a score based on the information inputted by the user. The score places the user into one of several risk categories graded from low to high risk. The intervention also provides feedback and specific advice on minimising risk based on another algorithm. The feedback content differs between online screening and feedback intervention programmes but usually includes statements about the person's estimated level of risk, how this estimated level of risk compares to the rest of the population (for example to the 'norm'), advice about what a person can do to reduce their alcohol and other drug use or level of risk, and the contact details of services or self-help support they may wish to access.

A number of researchers have studied the impact of online screening and feedback interventions on alcohol use (see Donoghue et al., 2014; Riper et al., 2014), and to a lesser extent drug use (Sinadinovic et al., 2012), with some reporting reductions in use as a consequence of the intervention. Many of these researchers have used randomised controlled trial designs, in which online screening and feedback interventions are compared to no intervention or screening only controls. The aim of these studies is to examine what effects these interventions have on alcohol and other drug use and related problems. In these studies, context and complexity are things to be controlled for, rather than things to be understood as co-constituting effects. This contributes to a sense that these interventions act in stable and consistent ways irrespective of the particularities of intervention users and the context in which the intervention is used. As with other digital health technologies, alcohol and other drug online screening and feedback interventions have not generally been analysed as 'sociocultural products' which play a 'role in configuring and enacting concepts and experiences of embodiment, selfhood and social relations in the context of medicine and public health' (Lupton, 2014, p. 1349). Very little work has critically examined the assumptions that online screening and feedback interventions make about alcohol and other drug use/users and problems, the qualitative experience of intervention recipients, or any unintended consequences that may arise. In this article, we examine these issues through an analysis of the content of one particular online screening and feedback intervention, as well as recipients' perceptions and experiences of the intervention.

Neoliberalism, complexity and enacting risk

While commentators have argued that online screening and feedback interventions have the potential to reach more people than face-to-face screening and feedback interventions (see Kypri et al., 2014), there are other possible implications of digitisation that are worth considering. The removal of the health professional from the traditional screening and feedback intervention process places even greater emphasis and responsibility on the individual using online screening and feedback interventions. We can therefore situate online screening and feedback interventions within an increasing tendency for neoliberal responses to be employed in relation to issues such as alcohol and other drug use (Zajdow & MacLean, 2014). Instead of being social problems that are subject to social controls and collectivist responses, neoliberalism has rebadged alcohol and other drug problems as problems of 'individual deficit and self-regulation' (Zajdow & MacLean, 2014, p. 524). Discourses of risk and self-management have become prominent (Moore & Fraser, 2006; Zajdow & MacLean, 2014). This rebranding is based on the logic that the inability to manage alcohol and other drug use (and by extension, the self) is a deficiency of the neoliberal subject that can be rectified through education and information about moderation (Zajdow & MacLean, 2014). Instead of the identification and management of alcohol and other drug problems being the responsibility of health professionals, online screening and feedback interventions are based on the assumption that when provided with 'scientific' information about their risk of alcohol and other drug problems and about what to do, individuals should be able to manage and seek help for their 'problems' by themselves. As a result, responsibility for, and agency over, problems are located within the individual, which can be experienced as empowering or disempowering (see Moore & Fraser, 2006). This placing of responsibility on the individual can also result in individuals being 'blamed for harm' (Rhodes, 2009, p. 194). Furthermore, it does not take into account the array of forces that may act to impede or facilitate risk management beyond the individual (Moore, 2004; Moore & Fraser, 2006; Rhodes, 2009).

Another related possible shortcoming of online screening and feedback interventions is their inability to account for complexity. While face-to-face screening and feedback interventions allow for the possibility of further discussion and clarification between health professionals and intervention recipients, recipients of online screening and feedback interventions typically have no opportunity to discuss their alcohol and other drug use in the context of their life circumstances, the situations in which their alcohol and other drug use occurs, and the reasons for their alcohol and other drug use. Instead, the experience of alcohol and other drug use is reduced to simple categories of risk that are communicated by means of generic feedback. Online screening and feedback interventions may be viewed as technologies for 'diagnosing risk as a disease state in and of itself' (Fosket, 2004, p. 294). As Fosket (2004) notes: 'within this model, we are all becoming ill because we are all, to varying degrees, at risk of something' (p. 294).

However, risk is far from value-neutral and self-evident (Lock, 1998) and there is the possibility that it may be constituted differently (Montelius & Nygren, 2014). Rather than viewing risk as 'an objective measurement of hazards or dangers' (p. 431), Montelius and Nygren (2014) view risk as performative, as 'something that is done' (p. 433) (and 'undone'), and entangled with the 'doing' of other things (such as gender, class, alcohol and other drug use). This 'doing risk' approach (Montelius & Nygren, 2014; Nygren, Öhman, & Olofsson, 2015) draws on notions of intersectionality and the performance of gender (Butler, 1993). Despite drawing on different theory, namely the work of Latour (2005) and Callon (1986), van Loon (2014) also argues for a performative understanding of risk in his discussion of 'cyber risk'. Unlike 'the constructionist perspective', in which risk is framed as a representation of the natural world (Brown, 2014), van Loon (2014) argues that 'risk is indistinguishable from the practices through which it comes into being' (p.447), and that it is mediated through networks of human and non-human actors. Following this argument, risk (or alcohol and other drug use for that matter) is therefore not stable but may emerge in different ways depending on the configuration of the network. However, risk is nested in a pre-existing hinterland (Law, 2004), which refers to 'the networks of relations between statements, practices, skills, objects and actors that are always already in place' (Dwyer & Moore, 2013, p. 204). This means that 'undoing' risk, or constituting risk in ways that don't conform to the dominant conceptualisation, can be difficult. The dominant hinterland in relation to risky alcohol and other drug use might be broadly characterised in terms of 'prevention science' (Toumborou, 2002), which has sought to develop an 'evidence base' around strategies to prevent alcohol and other drug problems (Duff, 2003). This prevention science hinterland may include national guidelines for safe use, public health messages and responses, drug education, screening tools, bio-medicine, neuroscience, neoliberalism and alcohol and other drug related epidemiology among other factors – all of which reinforce the notion of alcohol and other drugs as inherently risky irrespective of the way and setting in which they are used. Through repeated (re)enactment, the inherent riskiness of alcohol and other drug use becomes 'fact like', masking other possible ways in which alcohol and other drug use might be 'performed'.

'Expert' and 'lay' accounts of risk

The prevention science hinterland can be seen as producing 'expert' risk assessments, based on science (Beck, 1992). However, this may contrast with 'lay' risk assessments, which 'emerge from within the very cultural settings in which this risk behaviour takes place' and are managed as a 'fact of life' (Duff, 2003, p. 291). In the struggle between the 'rational' expert and 'functional' lay knowledge of risk, expert determinations of risk in relation to drug use often prevail (2003). Expert knowledge is considered 'objective' in contrast to lay knowledge, which is 'subjective' (Duff, 2003). However, Duff (2003) shows how young drug users may also come to distrust expert discourses of risk, viewing government-sponsored drug education campaigns, for instance, as exaggerating the risks and harms of alcohol and other drugs, and as preaching (Carroll, 2000). This may weaken the effectiveness of programmes and interventions employing expert notions of risky alcohol and other drug use. Duff (2003), like Foster and Heyman (2013), highlights the need to examine alcohol and other drug users' own perceptions and experiences of risk.

It is important to subject online screening and feedback interventions to critical analysis because assessing risk has potential implications for how people are viewed and view themselves. If risk discourses are about identifying and controlling pathologies concealed within the body (Lupton, 1995), then being diagnosed as 'at risk' may lead to 'an increased sense of unease and distrust with one's own body' (Fosket, 2004, p. 294). Being labelled as 'dependent' may come with a certain degree of stigma (Barry, McGinty, Pescosolido, & Goldman, 2014). Alternatively, a categorisation of risk may enable people to access health care and treatment more readily than if they were not identified as being at risk (Fosket, 2004).

Given the potential role of online screening and feedback interventions in the categorisation of risky alcohol and other drug use and users, in this article, we subject an online screening and feedback intervention to critical analysis. We explore how an online screening and feedback intervention enacts risk in relation to alcohol and other drug use/users, whether it accounts for complexity, and how alcohol and other drug users' accounts of risk compare to the way the expert risk assessment of the intervention characterises them.

Methods

In this article, we analyse the content of an online screening and feedback intervention, as well as the comments of people who used the intervention, as a way of examining how risky alcohol and other drug use/users are enacted in and through the intervention, and how these compare to intervention recipients' own accounts.

The intervention

The online screening and feedback intervention that is the focus of this article has been previously described (Wilson, Best, Savic, & Lubman, 2013) and was developed as an alternative treatment approach for adults who may not necessarily have sought help from a face-to-face alcohol and other drug service. Three of the authors of this article (Michael Savic, Fiona Barker and Dan Lubman) were involved in the development and ongoing improvement of the intervention. It was made available through the website of Turning Point, a national alcohol and other drug treatment, research and education organisation in Melbourne, Australia. The intervention can be completed on a computer, tablet or Smartphone that has internet access.

The screening component of the intervention was modelled on a screening tool that was developed for use in face-to-face alcohol and other drug treatment services in Victoria, Australia (Department of Health, 2013). It contains widely used standardised screening tools, which categorise people into risk categories based on their total scores (see Table 1). It also contains demographic questions (including age, gender, postcode) and questions on the types of substances people use, wellbeing and gambling. No contact details or email addresses are collected to preserve the anonymity of recipients of the intervention.

Table 1.   Screening tools and measures in the OSAFI.

Screening tool	Purpose	Score range	Risk categories
Q2 from the Alcohol, Tobacco & Substance Involvement Screening Test (ASSIST) (WHO ASSIST Working Group, 2002; Humeniuk et al., 2008)	Identify substances used in the past month	Not scored	N/A
10-item Alcohol Use Disorders Identification Test (AUDIT) (Babor, Higgins-Biddle, Saunders, & Monteiro, 2001)	Identifies risky alcohol use in the past year	0–40	Low risk = 1–7 Moderate risk = 8–15 High risk = 16–19 Dependence likely = 20+ (Babor et al., 2001)
11-item Drug Use Disorders Identification Test (DUDIT) (Berman, Bergman, Palmstierna, & Schlyter, 2003)	Identifies risky drug use (not including alcohol) in the past year	0–44	Low risk (male) = 1–5 Low risk (female) = 1 Harmful (male) = 6–24 Harmful (female) = 2–24 Dependence likely = 25+ (Berman et al., 2003)
10-item Kessler 10 (K10) (Kessler et al., 2002)	Identifies level of psychological distress in the past month	10–50	Little or no distress = 10–19 Mild distress = 20–24 Moderate distress = 25–29 High distress = 30+ (ABS, 2012)
3 Wellbeing items (quality of life, physical health, and psychological health) from the Australian Treatment Outcomes Profile (ATOP) (Ryan et al., 2014)	Rating of satisfaction with aspects of wellbeing in the past four weeks	0–10 for each item	Higher scores indicate higher satisfaction with wellbeing than lower scores. No thresholds or norms determined for Australia.
Problem Gambling Severity Index (PGSI) short-form (Ferris & Wynne, 2001; Volbert & Williams, 2012)	Identifies problematic and pathological gambling in the past year	0–9	Problematic and pathological gambling = 3+ (Volbert & Williams, 2012) *Note: Only included when the online screen was updated*

After recipients complete the screening component they are provided with automated feedback (see Appendix 1), which was devised based on guidelines from each of the respective screening tools and with input from alcohol and other drug clinicians. The automated feedback communicates the recipient's level of risk for each of the screening tools. A statement of where the person sits relative to other people who have used the intervention is provided for the Alcohol Use Disorders Identification Test (AUDIT), Drug Use Disorders Identification Test (DUDIT), Kessler 10 psychological distress scale (K10) and wellbeing items as a way of enabling comparison to 'similar' people. For tools where there is population level data available (such as the AUDIT and K10), normative feedback is also provided in the form of a statement about how the recipient's assessed level of risk compares to population statistics. This is thought to motivate behaviour change (Gaume et al., 2014). Further information about alcohol and other drug harms is also provided in the automated feedback. Finally, the automated feedback concludes with suggestions, links and contact details for further information and support that is commensurate with the level of risk. These predominantly consist of self-help information, online counselling, telephone helplines and face-to-face alcohol and other drug treatment services.

Data collection

Prior to beginning the intervention, participants were informed that advancing to the next screen was considered implied consent for data to be used for research purposes. Ethics approval was obtained for the use of intervention data via the Eastern Health Human Research Ethics Committee (11/06/2013, reference number LR85/1213). As well as collecting responses to each of the individual questions from the screening component of the intervention, data was collected on recipients' experience of the intervention via an optional survey at the end of the intervention. This asked a range of tick-box and rating type questions about where and when people used the intervention and how useful it was. There was also an open-ended question in which intervention participants were asked to describe their experience and perceptions of the intervention in their own words. This was initially worded 'Did you find the feedback and recommendations in your results page helpful?' and contained a 'Yes' or 'No' response, followed by an open text box for people to provide further comments. The question was later revised as part of a minor amendment to the intervention, and at the time of the research read: 'Do you have any recommendations/feedback on how we can improve the questionnaire?' Similarly, the question was followed by an open text box for people to enter their response. Responses were typically a sentence to a paragraph in length, and often contained participants' reflections on what they found helpful or unhelpful about the intervention, as well as how the intervention's assessment of risk compared to their own experiences and assessment of risk.

Participants

A total of 4041 people completed the online screen and feedback intervention between December 2012 and January 2015. People typically completed the intervention in their own homes or in other non-health care environments without the assistance of a health professional. In this article, we draw on data from the 489 intervention participants who completed the open-ended question in the optional survey about their experience of completing the intervention. The characteristics of this group of participants are outlined in Table 2. The most common ways participants reported hearing about the intervention were via an internet search (308, 63%), a case worker (28, 6%) or a friend (23, 5%).

Table 2. Participant characteristics.

Characteristic	Statistic
Gender (*n* = 489)	Female: 266 (54%)
Age (*n* = 488, <1% data missing)	<25: 72 (15%)
	25–39: 231 (47%)
	40+: 185 (38%)
Country of birth (*n* = 74, 85% data missing)	Born in Australia: 61 (82%)
Indigenous status (*n* = 489)	Aboriginal or Torres Strait Islander: 10 (2%)
Highest level of education (*n* = 489)	University: 183 (37%)
Employment status (*n* = 489)	Employed: 366 (75%)
Alcohol and other drug use in past month (*n* = 489)	Alcohol: 439 (80%)
	Cannabis: 180 (37%)
	Cocaine: 71 (15%)
	Amphetamines: 177 (36%)
	Inhalants: 28 (6%)
	Sedatives: 176 (36%)
	Hallucinogens: 59 (12%)
	Opioids: 89 (18%)
Alcohol and other drug problem severity according to AUDIT and DUDIT (*n* = 489)	Alcohol abstainers: 51 (10%)
	Alcohol low risk: 129 (26%)
	Alcohol moderate to high risk: 138 (28%)
	Alcohol dependence likely: 171 (35%)
	Drug abstainers: 218 (45%)
	Drug use low risk: 20 (4%)
	Drug use harmful: 116 (24%)
	Drug dependence likely: 135 (28%)
Ever accessed alcohol and other drug treatment (*n* = 489)	122 (25%)
Psychological distress (*n* = 489)	High psychological distress: 173 (35%)

Data analysis

We analysed the text from the automated feedback component of the intervention (detailed in Appendix 1) as well as the responses (*n* = 489) to the open-ended question about experiences and perceptions of the intervention. We extracted the participants' responses to the open-ended question from a database held by our organisation that contained all data from the intervention, which we imported into NVivo 10 (QSR International, 2012) along with the automated feedback text. We analysed the data using the inductive constant comparison method (Seale, 1999), in which data coding and analysis occur simultaneously in order to develop theoretically relevant concepts and themes from the data. As part of this process, the first author coded similar segments of text together to identify themes and their properties and to develop a coding framework. We were also interested in divergent or unique perspectives in order to foreground the range of experiences and tensions that can occur in relation to the intervention. The process of refining the coding framework was informed by our reading of the literature on alcohol and other drug use, risk, performativity and subjectivity. The way in which the online screening and feedback intervention enacted risk in relation to alcohol and other drug use/users, and how intervention recipients talked about their own alcohol and other drug use and level of risk, emerged as key themes. By comparing the intervention's risk assessment and recipients' own accounts of risk, we identified points of consistency and divergence. We use pseudonyms in this article when referring to intervention participants.

Findings

The intervention as the 'expert'

Many participants in our study thought that the intervention provided an expert and objective assessment of their risk of alcohol and other drug problems. Terms such as 'objective, 'unbiased', 'honest' and 'independent' were used to describe the feedback recipients received. For these people the intervention held up a 'mirror' to their lives and was considered to be 'the truth' or 'reality', or as Larry commented:

> The information helped me to review my honesty about my drug and alcohol use.

The assumption here is that the intervention held 'the objective and infallible truth', against which Larry could compare 'the honesty' of his own 'subjective' account of alcohol and other drug use. For these participants, the intervention created a sense of 'objectivity' and 'expertness' by being situated within the prevention science hinterland. It enabled participants to identify 'quantifiable' risks to health and wellbeing as a result of their alcohol and other drug use, through the use of screening tools. For instance, Marko commented that the screening tools:

> Lets me know the level of harm I am doing to myself.

Prior to starting the intervention, participants were presented with information on the screening tools contained within, and were provided with links to manuals and scientific articles related to the 'validation' of each. This helped establish the credibility of the online screening and feedback intervention from the outset as an 'evidence-based' intervention, which contains screening tools developed by 'experts', and which, therefore, provides 'expert risk assessment'. Indeed, Sandra, who was classified in the 'dependence likely' category, commented that the screening tools provided 'more evidence' of her drug problem. Other participants similarly commented on the screening tools as providing them with evidence of 'their situation', 'dependence', or 'addiction' or the absence of a 'problem'.

The automated feedback cited other high profile sources of prevention science. For instance, the intervention quoted the National Health and Medical Research Council's Australian Guidelines to Reduce Health Risks from Drinking (NHMRC, 2009). These 'evidence-based' and expert-developed guidelines specified how much an individual could safely drink to reduce the risk of short- and long-term alcohol harms, and also specified circumstances when 'not drinking alcohol may be the safest option'. Frank considered the feedback to be an:

> Unbiased commentary of my alcohol and drug consumption.

Like other participants, he evoked the sense that 'the expert' feedback provided was 'unbiased' in comparison to the partiality of other commentaries on his alcohol and other drug use.

The use of numbers, statistics and the quantification of risk, tended to bolster the objectivity and credibility of the intervention. Numeric rating scales are used throughout the screening component of the intervention, and one intervention participant noted how this increased the credibility of the system:

> The idea of a number on a scale is a good indicator of how severe a particular case may be.

The participants received a final 'risk' score based on their responses to questions in the screening tool. This score was an indicator of the level of risk and severity of alcohol and other drug problems they were experiencing. The intervention then provided feedback on how the user's risk rating compared to that of the general population. For instance Jane, whose alcohol use was categorised as high risk on the AUDIT, evoked this percentage in her comments about the intervention:

> '5% of the population drink at this level'. Holy shit, didn't realise my drinking was high risk – that was a real shock.

Jane's surprise at learning that her alcohol use was riskier than she had thought (and riskier than other peoples' drinking), according to the intervention, highlighted the potential effects of the use of numbers in shaping how people come to understand risk in the context of alcohol and other drug use. It also focuses our attention on what happens to lay accounts of risk in the presence of expert accounts.

Expert versus lay accounts

Just over a quarter of participants stated that 'the objective reality' which the intervention enacted carried more weight than their own perceptions of risk. For instance, Sally scored 12 on the AUDIT and was categorised in the moderate risk category for alcohol, and similarly scored 12 on the DUDIT, which placed her drug use in the harmful category. Sally commented that:

> Well I guess I wasn't sure if I had a problem or not and judging by the self test I do. It was indicated in more than one area.

Sally's uncertainty about whether her alcohol and other drug use was 'problematic' was overridden by the perceived certainty of the results of the online screening, which 'revealed' that her alcohol and other drug use was potentially harmful.

In over half of cases, participants reported that the intervention's assessment of risk confirmed their own understanding of the riskiness of their alcohol and other drug use. Some participants talked about the intervention as reinforcing 'what I already know', 'validating my own thoughts' and as 'confirming risk levels'. This group of participants problematised the intervention's assumption that people simply need information in order to moderate their alcohol and other drug use, as they already possessed information about the 'risks' associated with their alcohol and other drug use. Some participants noted that prior awareness of the prevention science literature and messages had shaped their responses to their risk assessment and associated information. As Sam said:

> [I] already knew most of the information as I researched and read a lot for my health and wellbeing and recovery issues, detoxification and finally side effects.

For these individuals, there was congruence between their 'lay' account of risk and the expert assessment.

However, in just under a quarter of cases, participants felt their assessment and understanding of the riskiness of alcohol and other drug use conflicted with the expert assessment and account. These individuals challenged the ways in which the intervention categorised their alcohol and other drug use as being risky, disregarding its context; that is the time, place and reasons they used alcohol or other drugs. For instance, Charlie was categorised as being in the 'harmful' drug use category but commented that:

> It's prescription drugs I am mostly on due to a car accident but it doesn't ask about which type of drug. For example is it recreational or prescription?

As Charlie's comments intimate, the screening tool cannot acknowledge his life history and the circumstances that have led to his drug use, the benefits he might derive in terms of coping after his accident, or the different reasons why people use drugs as it treats all drug use the same, reducing it to a single score and category.

Another manifestation of discontent with the inability of the tool to acknowledge the complexity of their alcohol and other drug use was its medicalisation of their alcohol and drug use as 'dependence'. For these participants, the intervention failed to take into account the reasons why they engaged in alcohol and other drug use, and in particular, the other risks it helped them minimise. For instance, Tom scored 14 on the DUDIT placing his drug use in the 'harmful' category, but he contested this categorisation. He argued that his cannabis use enabled him to deal with the stresses of everyday life:

> I only use cannabis, nothing else, which I find settles me and my anger down a fair bit as I stay stressed out most of the time daily.

Tom, along with several other participants argued that people could use drugs for therapeutic purposes, such as 'self-medicating' or 'self-managing' but there was no way the online screening tool could identify such use as there were no questions on why individuals used drugs, just questions on the quantity and frequency of use. The way in which the intervention disregarded the context of Tom's cannabis use and classified it as high risk is consistent with prevention science's 'acontextual' enactment of cannabis and its effects (Duff, 2003). Other participants commented on the recreational and social reasons they used alcohol and other drugs. Sarah, whose alcohol use was categorised by the intervention as 'moderate risk' and whose drug use was considered to be 'harmful', pointed out that the intervention:

> ... didn't address the fact that substances make me feel good and I want to keep doing them.

Indeed, there are no questions in the standardised screening tools that ask about pleasure, nor is there acknowledgement of the potential for the positive impacts of alcohol and other drug use in the automated feedback text.

Some participants noted the ways in which the online screening and feedback intervention drew on conventional wisdom that links alcohol and other drug use to poor physical health, mental health and quality of life (see Laudet, 2011). They noted that the intervention's feedback in relation to quality of life was based solely on drug use, as it stated:

It is possible that your substance use is affecting your psychological health, your physical health and even your quality of life.

As Anna noted, this completely failed to consider the impact of other aspects of her life. The intervention placed Anna in the harmful drug use category as well as in the experiencing 'mild psychological distress' category. Anna agreed that she was experiencing 'psychological distress' but argued that this 'distress' was not a product of her drug use but of other factors in her life:

> Questions [in the online screening tool] did not ask why I was feeling those things. I have actually cut down drug use to once in the last 3 months, yet feel depressed about my husband having an affair. This tool is too primitive to separate these things.

Some participants commented negatively on the generalised nature of the automatic feedback, which was not particularly tailored to their specific experiences. Participants described it as 'stock standard', 'not personalised' and 'general'. Tony said that the experience of using the intervention was:

> ... more like talking to a machine that gives you pre-planned answers, like Chinese cookies.

Some participants felt that the intervention lacked a human or personal quality and therefore could not provide a personalised response, nor acknowledge the complexity of alcohol and other drug use. Jim, for instance, was categorised as likely to be dependent on alcohol and other drugs and scored the highest possible psychological distress score on the K10. While completing the intervention provided information, it did not provide the help he desired, and this is evident in his comment, in which he also included his phone number:

> I need someone to contact me.

Fragile subjects in need of professional help

While most of the participants liked the range of help and support options provided in the automated feedback, some recipients felt the advice provided was too focused on professional solutions to addressing risk. For instance, Gemma's alcohol and other drug use were categorised as low risk by the intervention but she was still advised to seek expert help. She commented that:

> It advised me to seek help when there was no risk level. I know AOD [alcohol and other drug] services would baulk at the idea of someone with this low level risk contacting them and it came across as a bit clinical/cold/labelling/medicalised in its process of advice.

Some participants rejected the assumption underlying the intervention that problematic alcohol and drug use could only be managed using expert advice and guidance. They wanted to manage risk themselves. For example Dino, who the intervention categorised as likely to be drug dependent, wanted more information on how he could manage his use himself:

Mostly recommended to call a number and really does not give me a chance to work with myself and try to get drug free on my own hand. More suggestions and more information how to stop using drugs all by yourself would be great.

Dino's comments might be seen as fitting within a neoliberal framework of self-management and indeed, the prevention science hinterland, but his desire or ability to self-manage was not acknowledged within the intervention, which suggested that he seek professional support.

Discussion

Our analysis of the way in which an online screening and feedback intervention enacts risk in relation to alcohol and other drug use/users suggests that interventions, like online screening and feedback interventions, act in ways that may not be intended or routinely considered by prevention science researchers. By drawing on existing prevention science resources, knowledge and practices, such as standardised screening tools, national guidelines, algorithms and quantification into categories of risk, the online screening and feedback intervention cultivated a sense of 'expertness' and objectivity.

However, Dwyer & Fraser's (2015) critical analysis of addiction screening and diagnostic tools highlights the tenuousness of validity claims these tools make and shows that they 'make certainty where there is none' through scientific validation techniques (p. 1). Lupton and Jutel (2015) also illustrate how self-diagnosis applications (apps) draw on algorithms and discourses of healthism to cultivate a sense of authority, power and objectivity, which is undermined by their own disclaimers about not being substitutes for medical practitioner diagnosis.

The use of numbers was implicated in the sense of authority and validity that the online screening and feedback intervention cultivated. The complexity of peoples' alcohol and other drug use experiences were reduced to a simple number, which provided 'evidence' of a person's level of risk. Numbers carry weight because they are 'eminently mobile, decontextualised, and fact like' (Fosket, 2004, p. 297), even though the meaning of numbers are subject to interpretation and are the result of a number of conscious decisions. The development of different systems of cut-off scores, used to allocate people into categories of risk on the same screening tool (Australian Bureau of Statistics [ABS], 2012), illustrates this and draws the 'fact like' appearance of the online screening and feedback intervention into question.

In unsettling the 'objectivity' of screening tools, Dwyer and Fraser argue that such tools 'actively participate in the creation of social objects and social groups, and in shaping affected individuals and their opportunities' (Dwyer & Fraser, 2015, p. 1). Similarly, our analysis highlights the role of the online screening and feedback intervention in how intervention recipients come to know themselves as risky alcohol and other drug users or not. This point is particularly borne out in the first of the three modes of interaction between expert and alcohol and other drug user accounts of risk that we identified.

Consistent with Duff's (2003) discussion, the first mode of interaction involved the expert risk assessment overshadowing alcohol and other drug users' own accounts of risk and being considered a more 'valid' assessment of risk. Intervention recipients' understandings of themselves, their alcohol and other drug use experiences and bodies are likely to be altered in the process of deferring to the expert risk assessment, particularly when the intervention categorised their alcohol and other drug use as riskier than they had otherwise thought. The shock and despair that some intervention recipients expressed when faced with diverging accounts of risk and the discovery of 'being a risky alcohol and other drug user' reiterates the role of digital health technologies in co-constituting subjectivities and experiences of the body (Lupton, 2014). This mode of interaction also highlights the potential for online screening and feedback interventions to encourage anxiety and/or distrust of one's own assessment of risk, which may further enshrine the dominance of an expert prevention science discourse about alcohol and other drug risk (Duff, 2003). Deferring to the expert risk assessment discourse rather than trusting one's own risk assessment may also act counter to the neoliberal framework of self-monitoring and regulation.

The second mode of interaction between alcohol and other drug user and expert accounts of risk was where the intervention's assessment 'validated' alcohol and other drug user's own pre-existing risk assessment. Some of the intervention recipients whose comments conformed to this mode of interaction had been exposed to prevention science messages and information. These intervention recipients might be seen as embracing prevention science's focus on leading a healthy lifestyle (Burrows, Nettleton, & Bunton, 1995) and the neoliberal imperative of self-care (Moore & Fraser, 2006). The fact that intervention recipients sought out the online screening and feedback intervention might further indicate their possible openness to a neoliberal subjectivity, and/or reflect their willingness to trust digital health technologies in general, given their increasing avail-ability (Lupton, 2014). This group also problematises the binary opposition between expert and lay accounts of risk in that their comments do not conform to the contextua-lised and 'subjective' lay accounts of risk previously discussed. Instead, they valorise the expert assessment of risk provided by the intervention, and reiterate the dominance and reach of the prevention science paradigm.

Finally, the participants for whom the intervention's determination of risk did not accurately reflect their own experience of alcohol and other drug use and risk, might be seen as resisting 'expert' prevention science enactments of alcohol and other drug use as inherently risky. Given the lack of questions in the intervention on the context of drug use and the potential benefits such as pleasure or feeling better, the intervention could not, and showed no capacity to, deal with nuanced understandings of pleasure and harm, which highlight that harms may not be typically experienced without pleasure and vice versa (Pennay, 2015). The participants in our study commented on the multiplicity of possible realities and effects that can be associated with alcohol and other drug use, few of which were asked about in the screening tools and thus were not accounted for in providing feedback. Far from 'passive recipients of information', these participants actively and critically engaged with risk information (Alaszewski, 2005, p. 104). They provided nuanced and contextualised accounts of the multiple reasons why people engage in alcohol and other drug use, and took issue with the reduction of the complex-ity of their experiences to simple categories of risk; an act that re-enacts alcohol and other drug use as singularly and predictably dangerous or harmful, to the exclusion of any benefits or other effects. Their accounts encourage us to view alcohol and other drug use and risk in contextualised ways (Keane, 2009). For instance, Rhodes (2009) focuses attention on the 'risk environment', which 'envisages drug harms as a product of the social situations and environments in which individuals participate' (p. 193). Like Duff (2007), we might consider alcohol and other drug use and risk as embedded in a complex assemblage of interacting and co-constituting relations, actors, use-values, practices and settings. When alcohol and other drug use is isolated from this complex assemblage of forces, our understanding of people's experience of alcohol and other drug use and risk is limited.

Our analysis also highlights the way in which the intervention medicalises risk and enacts recipients as fragile and in need of professional help. It is here that the tension between neoliberalism and the expert prevention science discourse is most explicit. On the one hand, the intervention assumes that recipients are neoliberal subjects who are capable of managing risk and changing their alcohol and other drug use when provided with feedback on their level of risk. However, the advice provided to intervention recipients overwhelmingly points people in the direction of professional support options rather than self-help. Lupton and Jutel (2015) note a similar tension in relation to self-diagnosis apps. These apps configure people as 'empowered consumers of health information' (p. 133), but by encouraging people to seek further advice from medical practitioners they place clear limits on people's capabilities and empowerment.

Given the tensions and multiple modes of interaction with the 'expertness' of the online screening and feedback intervention outlined, we suggest that online screening and feedback interventions should ideally be flexible enough to accommodate a diversity of modes of lay-expert risk assessment interaction, the subjectivities that people subscribe too – whether these conform to neoliberal ideals or not – and the complexities of alcohol and other drug use and risk. As numerous alcohol and other drug online screening and feedback interventions have been developed, often with more sophisticated functionality than the intervention we have discussed in this article (see HAGA, 2015), there are likely to be some that exemplify these ideals.

Online screening and feedback interventions may be better positioned to acknowledge complexity and context if they ask questions about the reasons, time, place and meanings of alcohol and other drug use and risk. However, online screening and feedback interventions may have difficulty in dealing with this sort of contextual data and complexity, especially if the data is qualitative. Algorithms may not be able to compute or adequately factor qualitative data into risk assessment. If context was elicited through quantitative data it would presumably require numerous different algorithms to account for all possible scenarios, and even then the degree to which it would be able to accurately 'account for all permutations' is doubtful. Consistent with other research (Klein et al., 2010), this is where we feel human contact may be helpful.

One of the ways in which online screening and feedback interventions might become more useful, particularly for those who are shocked by results or those whose own accounts of risk do not conform to the intervention's expert risk assessment, would be to provide greater opportunity for intervention users' own accounts of risk and risk management to be heard. For example, at the beginning or end of an online screening and feedback intervention, intervention users could be asked to comment on their alcohol and other drug use experiences and own accounts of risk, which they would then be able to compare with the intervention's assessment of risk. They could then be provided with the option of engaging in web chat with a counsellor instantaneously in order to discuss any divergence in accounts of risk, as a way to resolve this and better account for alcohol and other drug related pleasure and benefits and the complexities of alcohol and other drug use. This is consistent with a study of the content and functionality preferences of visitors to alcohol and other drug websites, which found that being able to ask a question was one of the most common interactive features that visitors endorsed as being important (Klein et al., 2010).

Similarly, intervention users could be invited to share strategies they have employed to manage alcohol and other drug related risk, which could then be made available to other intervention recipients as part of the automated feedback. This kind of 'see what other people have done to manage their alcohol and other drug use' capacity would act as another source of self-help information for people who find a neoliberal subjectivity empowering. One example of this is evident in the 'Don't Bottle it Up' online screening and feedback intervention in which people are invited to share their 'experiences, thoughts and tips with others who are thinking about their drinking' in one section of the website (HAGA, 2015). The inclusion of online self-help tools, such as self-help strategies, drink-diaries, plans for reducing consumption and links to additional information may provide more options for self-management, which users of alcohol and other drug websites may desire (Klein et al., 2010). The problem that researchers may encounter when greater options for drawing on lay accounts and sharing recipients' own risk management strategies is the risk that these strategies do not conform to, or even contradict, prevention science 'evidence'. Many institutions would presumably be concerned about the risk to themselves of proliferating 'non-evidence-based' material that they may see as 'harmful'. This is where further research to understand alcohol and other drug users' lived experiences and strategies for risk management would be useful. Using a researcher or clinician to moderate risk strategies shared by recipients may also mitigate this risk, although this still reinforces the expertness of the intervention. Ensuring the language used in automated feedback is not paternalistic, as well as pointing out the limitations of screening tools and of the expert prevention science enactment of risk, may also be useful.

This analysis is restricted to the content of one online screening and feedback intervention. Different online screening and feedback interventions are likely to have different content and functionality, which may impact on recipient experiences and enactments of risk. Our analysis was also limited to recipient comments provided in response to an open-ended question in an optional survey at the end of the intervention. The majority of intervention recipients did not respond to the open-ended question, and thus may have had different experiences of the intervention and different accounts of risk to those participants who did respond. Analysing responses to the open-ended survey question meant that we could not probe further as we might have done had we interviewed intervention users. For instance, we do not know how recipients actually used the automated feedback information they were provided with. Research employing in-depth qualitative interviews with users of online screening and feedback interventions is likely to generate rich data and further insights about how risk and subjectivities are performed and negotiated through online interventions.

Conclusion

Concern about the effectiveness of digital health technologies has relegated their assumptions and logics to the background (Lupton, 2014). In making the assumptions and workings of an online screening and feedback intervention visible, along with the experiences of intervention recipients, we have shown how the intervention is implicated in the enactment of risky alcohol and other drug use/users. As our analysis suggests, and as others have noted (Dwyer & Fraser, 2015), interventions and tools can shape how alcohol and other drug users understand themselves and their experiences of alcohol and other drug use and risk. Drawing on prevention science discourses about the inherent riskiness of alcohol and other drug use and neoliberal discourses of individual responsibility, the intervention is established as providing an authoritative and objective assessment of risk, which sometimes overshadows recipients' own accounts of risk. However, the nuanced and contextualised accounts of intervention recipients' who didn't agree with the intervention's 'expert' assessment of risk highlight how risk in relation to alcohol and other drug use might be 'done' differently; how it might emerge differently in different situations and with different effects, and therefore provoke different responses. We suggest that subjecting online alcohol and other drug tools and interventions to critical analysis may be a useful step in unsettling problematic assumptions about alcohol and other drug use/ users and risk and more sensitively attending to complex alcohol and other drug use experiences.

Acknowledgements

We would like to thank all the participants who kindly shared their experiences of using the intervention with us. We would also like to thank the anonymous reviewers for their useful comments, as well as Amy Pennay for her helpful feedback on an earlier draft of this article.

Disclosure statement

No potential conflict of interest was reported by the authors.

References

Australian Bureau of Statistics. (2012). *Information paper: Use of the Kessler Psychological Distress Scale in ABS health surveys, Australia, 2007-08*. Canberra: Author.

Alaszewski, A. (2005). Risk communication: Identifying the importance of social context. *Health, Risk & Society, 7*(2), 101–105. doi:10.1080/13698570500148905

Babor, T. F., & Higgins-Biddle, J. C. (2001). *Brief intervention for hazardous and harmful drinking: A manual for use in primary care*. Geneva: World Health Organization.

Babor, T. F., Higgins-Biddle, J. C., Saunders, J. B., & Monteiro, M. G. (2001). *AUDIT: The Alcohol Use Disorders Identification Test guidelines for use in primary care – second edition*. Geneva: World Health Organization.

Babor, T. F., McRee, B. G., Kassebaum, P. A., Grimaldi, P. L., Ahmed, K., & Bray, J. (2007). Screening, brief intervention, and referral to treatment (SBIRT): Toward a public health approach to the management of substance abuse. *Substance Abuse, 28*(3), 7–30. doi:10.1300/J465v28n03_03

Barry, C. L., McGinty, E. E., Pescosolido, B. A., & Goldman, H. H. (2014). Stigma, discrimination, treatment effectiveness, and policy: Public views about drug addiction and mental illness. *Psychiatric Services, 65*(10), 1269–1272. doi:10.1176/appi.ps.201400140

Beck, U. (1992). *Risk society: Towards a new modernity* (Vol. 17). London: Sage.

Berman, A. H., Bergman, H., Palmstierna, T., & Schlyter, F. (2003). *DUDIT: The Drug Use Disorders Identification Test manual version 1.0*. Stockholm: Department of Clinical Neuroscience, Karolinska Institutet.

Brown, P. (2014). Risk and social theory: The legitimacy of risks and risk as a tool of legitimation. *Health, Risk & Society, 16*(5), 391–397. doi:10.1080/13698575.2014.937678

Bunton, R. (2001). Knowledge, embodiment and neo-liberal drug policy. *Contemporary Drug Problems, 28*, 221. doi:10.1177/009145090102800204

Burrows, R., Nettleton, S., & Bunton, R. (1995). Sociology and health promotion: Health, risk and consumption under late modernism. In R. Burrows, S. Nettleton, & R. Bunton (Ed.), *The sociology of health promotion: Critical analyses of consumption, lifestyle and risk* (pp. 1–12). London and New York, NY: Routeledge.

Butler, J. (1993). *Bodies that matter: On the discursive limits of "sex"*. New York, NY: Routledge.

Callon, M. (1986). Some elements of a sociology of translation: Domestication of the scallops and the fishermen of St. Brieuc Bay. In J. Law (Ed.), *Power, action and belief: A new sociology of knowledge?* (pp. 196–233)). London: Routledge.

Carroll, T. (2000). *Illicit drugs: Research to aid in the development of strategies to target young people*. Sydney: Blue Moon Research and Planning.

Department of Health. (2013). *The adult AOD screening and assessment instrument: Clinician guide*. Melbourne: State Government of Victoria.

Donoghue, K., Patton, R., Phillips, T., Deluca, P., & Drummond, C. (2014). The effectiveness of electronic screening and brief intervention for reducing levels of alcohol consumption: A systematic review and meta-analysis. *Journal of Medical and Internet Research*, *16*(6), e142. doi:10.2196/jmir.3193

Duff, C. (2003). The importance of culture and context: Rethinking risk and risk management in young drug using populations. *Health, Risk & Society*, *5*(3), 285–299. doi:10.1080/13698570310001606987

Duff, C. (2007). Towards a theory of drug use contexts: Space, embodiment and practice. *Addiction Research & Theory*, *15*(5), 503–519. doi:10.1080/16066350601165448

Dwyer, R., & Fraser, S. (2015). Addiction screening and diagnostic tools: 'Refuting'and 'unmasking' claims to legitimacy. *International Journal of Drug Policy*, *26*(12), 1189–1197. doi:10.1016/j.drugpo.2015.08.016

Dwyer, R., & Moore, D. (2013). Enacting multiple methamphetamines: The ontological politics of public discourse and consumer accounts of a drug and its effects. *International Journal of Drug Policy*, *24*(3), 203–211. doi:10.1016/j.drugpo.2013.03.003

Ferris, J., & Wynne, H. (2001). *The Canadian Problem Gambling Index final report*. Ottawa: Canadian Centre on Substance Abuse.

Fosket, J. (2004). Constructing 'high-risk women': The development and standardization of a breast cancer risk assessment tool. *Science, Technology, & Human Values*, *29*(3), 291–313. doi:10.1177/0162243904264960

Foster, J., & Heyman, B. (2013). Drinking alcohol at home and in public places and the time framing of risks. *Health, Risk & Society*, *15*(6–7), 511–524. doi:10.1080/13698575.2013.839779

Gaume, J., McCambridge, J., Bertholet, N., & Daeppen, J.-B. (2014). Mechanisms of action of brief alcohol interventions remain largely unknown – A narrative review. *Frontiers in Psychiatry*, *5*, 108. doi:10.3389/fpsyt.2014.00108

HAGA. (2015). Don't bottle it up. Retrieved May 13, 2015, from https://dontbottleitup.org.uk/

Humeniuk, R., Ali, R., Babor, T. F., Farrell, M., Formigoni, M. L., Jittiwutikarn, J., ... Simon, S. (2008). Validation of the alcohol, smoking and substance involvement screening test (ASSIST). *Addiction*, *103*(6), 1039–1047. doi:10.1111/j.1360-0443.2007.02114.x

Keane, H. (2009). Intoxication, harm and pleasure: An analysis of the Australian National Alcohol Strategy. *Critical Public Health*, *19*(2), 135–142. doi:10.1080/09581590802350957

Kessler, R. C., Andrews, G., Colpe, L. J., Hiripi, E., Mroczek, D. K., Normand, S. L., ... Zaslavsky, A. M. (2002). Short screening scales to monitor population prevalences and trends in non-specific psychological distress. *Psychological Medicine*, *32*(06), 959–976. doi:10.1017/S0033291702006074

Klein, B., White, A., Kavanagh, D., Shandley, K., Kay-Lambkin, F., Proudfoot, J., ... Young, R. (2010). Content and functionality of alcohol and other drug websites: Results of an online survey. *Journal of Medical Internet Research*, *12*(5), e51. doi:10.2196/jmir.1449

Kypri, K., Vater, T., Bowe, S. J., Saunders, J. B., Cunningham, J. A., Horton, N. J., & McCambridge, J. (2014). Web-based alcohol screening and brief intervention for university students: A randomized trial. *Jama*, *311*(12), 1218–1224. doi:10.1001/jama.2014.2138

Latour, B. (2005). *Reassembling the social*. Oxford: Oxford University Press.

Laudet, A. B. (2011). The case for considering quality of life in addiction research and clinical practice. *Addiction Science & Clinical Practice*, *6*(1), 44.

Law, J. (2004). *After method: Mess in social science research*. London and New York, NY: Routledge.

Lock, M. (1998). Breast cancer: Reading the omens. *Anthropology Today*, *14*, 7–16. doi:10.2307/2783351

Lupton, D. (1995). *The imperative of health: Public health and the regulated body*. London: Sage.

Lupton, D. (2014). Critical perspectives on digital health technologies. *Sociology Compass*, *8*(12), 1344–1359. doi:10.1111/soc4.12226

Lupton, D., & Jutel, A. (2015). 'It's like having a physician in your pocket!' A critical analysis of self-diagnosis smartphone apps. *Social Science & Medicine*, *133*, 128–135. doi:10.1016/j.socscimed.2015.04.004

McCambridge, J., & Cunningham, J. A. (2014). The early history of ideas on brief interventions for alcohol. *Addiction*, *109*(4), 538–546. doi:10.1111/add.12458

Montelius, E., & Nygren, K. G. (2014). 'Doing' risk, 'doing' difference: Towards an understanding of the intersections of risk, morality and taste. *Health, Risk and Society*, *16*(5), 431–443. doi:10.1080/13698575.2014.934207

Moore, D. (2004). Governing street-based injecting drug users: A critique of heroin overdose prevention in Australia. *Social Science & Medicine*, *59*(7), 1547–1557. doi:10.1016/j.socscimed.2004.01.029

Moore, D., & Fraser, S. (2006). Putting at risk what we know: Reflecting on the drug-using subject in harm reduction and its political implications. *Social Science & Medicine*, *62*(12), 3035–3047. doi:10.1016/j.socscimed.2005.11.067

NHMRC. (2009). *Australian guidelines to reduce health risks from drinking alcohol*. Canberra: Commonwealth of Australia.

Nygren, G. K., Öhman, S., & Olofsson, A. (2015). Doing and undoing risk: The mutual constitution of risk and heteronormativity in contemporary society. *Journal of Risk Research*, 1–15. doi:10.1080/13669877.2015.1088056

Pennay, A. (2015). 'What goes up must go down': An exploration of the relationship between drug-related pleasure and harm experienced by a sample of regular 'party drug' users. *Drugs: Education, Prevention, and Policy*, 1–8. doi:10.3109/09687637.2015.1016398

QSR International. (2012). NVivo qualitative data analysis software (Version 10).

Rhodes, T. (2009). Risk environments and drug harms: A social science for harm reduction approach. *International Journal of Drug Policy*, *20*(3), 193–201. doi:10.1016/j.drugpo.2008.10.003

Riper, H., Blankers, M., Hadiwijaya, H., Cunningham, J., Clarke, S., & Wiers, R. (2014). Effectiveness of guided and unguided low-Intensity internet interventions for adult alcohol misuse: A meta-analysis. *PLoS ONE*, *9*(6), e99912. doi:10.1371/journal.pone.0099912

Ryan, A., Holmes, J., Hunt, V., Dunlop, A., Mammen, K., Holland, R., ... Lintzeris, N. (2014). Validation and implementation of the Australian treatment outcomes profile in specialist drug and alcohol settings. *Drug and Alcohol Review*, *33*(1), 33–42. doi:10.1111/dar.12083

Seale, C. (1999). *The quality of qualitative research*. London: Sage.

Sinadinovic, K., Wennberg, P., & Berman, A. H. (2012). Targeting problematic users of illicit drugs with Internet-based screening and brief intervention: A randomized controlled trial. *Drug and Alcohol Dependence*, *126*(1–2), 42–50. doi:10.1016/j.drugalcdep.2012.04.016

Toumborou, J. (2002). *Drug prevention strategies: A developmental settings approach prevention research evaluation report (number 2)*. Melbourne: The Drug Prevention Network.

van Loon, J. (2014). Remediating risk as matter-energy-information-flows of avian influenza and BSE. *Health, Risk & Society*, *16*(5), 444–458. doi:10.1080/13698575.2014.936833

Volbert, R. A., & Williams, R. J. (2012). *Developing a short form of the PGSI: Report to the Gambling Commission*. Great Britain: Gemini Research.

WHO ASSIST Working Group. (2002). The Alcohol, Smoking and Substance Involvement Screening Test (ASSIST): Development, reliability and feasibility. *Addiction*, *97*, 1183–1194. doi:10.1046/j.1360-0443.2002.00185.x

Wilson, A. S., Best, D. W., Savic, M., & Lubman, D. I. (2013). Online screening for alcohol and other drug problems: An acceptable method for accessing help. *The Medical Journal of Australia*, *199*(3), 170–170. doi:10.5694/mja13.10219

Zajdow, G., & MacLean, S. (2014). 'I just drink for that tipsy stage': Young adults and embodied management of alcohol use. *Contemporary Drug Problems*, *41*(4), 522–535. doi:10.1177/0091450914567123

Appendix 1: Automated feedback text

Your Results

ALCOHOL

Your score for the drinking assessment is xxx out of a possible score of 40, where higher scores indicate higher levels of risk of harm from drinking.

Score	Feedback
0	This indicates that you have not drunk alcohol in the last year.
1–7	Based on your answers, this result suggests that your current drinking level is **low risk**. Around 80% of the Australian population drink at this level, while 29% of people who recently used this screen got a similar score. If your drinking increases or you start to notice problems you may like to repeat this screen to see if your risk has changed. *Click here for more information.*
8–15	Based on your answers, this result suggests that your current drinking level is **moderate risk** and you may be at risk of an alcohol related illness or injury. Around 80% of the Australian population drinks less than you, while 20% of people who recently used this screen got a similar score. *Click here for more information.*
16–19	Based on your answers, this result suggests that your current drinking level is **high risk** and you are at risk of an alcohol related illness or injury. Around 96% of the Australian population drinks less than you, while 11% of people who recently used this screen got a similar score. *Click here for more information.*
20+	Based on your answers, this result suggests that your current drinking level is **very high risk** and that you might be **dependent** on alcohol. Around 98% of the Australian population drinks less than you, while 40% of people who recently used this screen got a similar score. *Click here for more information.*

DRUGS

Your score for the drugs-other-than-alcohol assessment is xxx out of a possible score of 44, where higher scores indicate higher levels of risk of harm from drug use.

Score	Feedback
0	This indicates that you have not used drugs in the last year.
Male = 1–5 Female = 1	Based on your answers, this result suggests that your current patterns of substance use are **low risk**. Around 53% of people who recently used this screen got a similar score. *Click here for more information.*
Male 6–24 Female 2–24	Based on your answers, this result suggests that your current patterns of substance use may be **harmful**. Around 22% of people who recently used this screen got a similar score. *Click here for more information.*
>24	Based on your answers, this result suggests that your drug use patterns are **harmful to your health** and that you may be **dependent**. Around 25% of people who recently used this screen got a similar score. *Click here for more information.*

ASSIST score > 0:
Your answers indicate that you have used the following drugs within the last month:

(1) [insert list of each drug type where response was >0 'never']

Click here for more information.

If score of 3+ to gambling questions:

GAMBLING

You have indicated that gambling may be causing problems in your life. *Click here for more information.*

PSYCHOLOGICAL DISTRESS

Your score for the psychological distress assessment is xxx out of a possible score of 50, where higher scores indicate higher levels of distress.

Score	Feedback
10–19	This score suggests you are experiencing little or no psychological distress. Around 70% of Australians have a similar level of distress, while around 30% of people who recently used this screen got a similar score.
20–24	This score suggests you are experiencing mild psychological distress. Around 20% of Australians have a similar level of distress, while 16% of people who recently used this screen got a similar score.
25–29	This score suggests you are experiencing moderate psychological distress. Around 7% of Australians have a similar level of distress, while around 17% of people who recently used this screen got a similar score.
30+	This score suggests you are experiencing high psychological distress which indicates a very high likelihood of an anxiety and/or depressive disorder. Around 3% of Australians have a similar level of distress, while around 36% of people who recently used this screen got a similar score.

WELLBEING

Psychological

You rated your **psychological health** to be xx out of 10, where higher scores indicate better psychological health. The average psychological health rating amongst people who have recently completed this screen is 4.5. This means that you are **above/below** the average.

Physical

You rated your **physical health** to be xx out of 10, where higher scores indicate better physical health. The average physical health rating amongst people who have recently completed this screen is 5.6. This means that you are **above/below** the average.

Quality of Life

You rated your **quality of life** to be xx out of 10, where higher scores indicate better quality of life. The average quality of life rating amongst people who have recently completed this screen is 4.9. This means that you are **above/below** the average. It is possible that your substance use is affecting your psychological health, your physical health and even your quality of life.

What can I do?

If any of your scores suggest that your substance use is at a risky level of harm, or that you are experiencing poor mental health and wellbeing, we recommend that you seek professional support to help you manage your problems.

Substance Use Problems

You can talk to a specialist substance counsellor either on the phone or online to discuss this further and to obtain referral for additional help if you want. Counsellors can provide confidential advice and guidance about the most appropriate support for your needs. For help with alcohol or other drugs we recommend:
DirectLine (1 800 888 236)

Provides telephone-based confidential alcohol and drug counselling and referral.
Counselling Online www.counsellingonline.org.au

Provides live online text-based counselling, information and referral for alcohol and other drug issues.
If you would like additional self-help advice, you may find the following websites useful:

JustAskUs	http://www.justaskus.org.au/
	Online assessments and self-help information about alcohol and other drugs.
Australian Drug Foundation	http://www.druginfo.adf.org.au/drug-facts/drug-information
	Facts and resources about alcohol and other drugs.

Mental Health Problems

If you need immediate help please call Lifeline:
Lifeline (13 11 14)
There are also online and telephone support options for mental health and we recommend:
Mental Health Online
www.anxietyonline.org.au
Beyond Blue (1 300 22 4636)
www.beyondblue.org.au
Telephone support and web chat

Mensline (1 300 78 99 78)
www.mensline.org.au
Telephone, online and video support
MindSpot (1 800 61 44 34)
www.mindspot.org.au
Online and telephone treatment for anxiety and depression
MindHealthConnect
www.mindhealthconnect.org.au
Factsheets and links to services and resources.

Alternatively, you can contact your GP to discuss how you feel. Your GP will refer you to a service that best meets your needs and give you information on the impacts on your health. If you would like access to an alcohol and drug service in your local area, have a look at the help section at the bottom of the page. They will offer help and advice and refer you to a specialist if that is your choice.

Need help?

If you need more information on services available in your area, select your state or territory below to find a listing of services available to you or look at this website **www2. betterhealth.vic.gov.au/saywhen/gethelp** for links to other services.

More Information

AUDIT Score 1–7

Based on your responses, you do not need to change your current drinking level as you do not exceed the recommended drinking guidelines. To find out more information on what the recommended Australian drinking levels are and what a standard drink is, please click on the links to information from the Australian Drug Foundation. We also recommend the SayWhen website, which has a range of tools and calculators to help you make decisions about your drinking.

How can I avoid risks from drinking?
To minimise your risk of harm from drinking, the National Health and Medical Research Council of Australia recommends the following guidelines:

For healthy men and women:

(1) drinking **no more than two standard drinks on any day** reduces the lifetime risk of harm from alcohol-related disease or injury
(2) drinking **no more than four standard drinks on a single occasion** reduces the risk of alcohol-related injury arising from that occasion.

Not drinking alcohol is the safest option if you:

(3) drive or operate heavy machinery
(4) are pregnant, planning a pregnancy or breastfeeding

(5) are under 18 years of age

Not drinking alcohol may also be the safest option if you:

(1) are taking other medications or drugs
(2) have a history of brain injury or liver disease

Please check with your doctor if you are not sure.

AUDIT Score 8–15

Based on your responses, you could think about monitoring your drinking behaviour and identify ways to reduce your drinking to low risk levels. To find out more information on what the recommended Australian drinking levels are and what a standard drink is, please click on the highlighted links to information from the Australian Drug Foundation. We also recommend the SayWhen website where you can find more information on the effects of drinking and tools to further assess your drinking and assist you with problems you may be having with your drinking.

Here are some tips you might like to try:

(1) Keep a record of when and where you tend to drink alcohol – this can help you to avoid problem areas.
(2) Have a couple of alcohol-free nights a week.
(3) Try activities that are less likely to involve alcohol, such as going to a movie.
(4) Eat before you drink and while you are drinking.
(5) Alternate your drinks by making every other drink a non-alcoholic one.

How can I avoid risks from drinking?
To minimise your risk of harm from drinking, the National Health and Medical Research Council of Australia recommends the following guidelines:

For healthy men and women:

(6) drinking **no more than two standard drinks on any day** reduces the lifetime risk of harm from alcohol-related disease or injury
(7) drinking **no more than four standard drinks on a single occasion** reduces the risk of alcohol-related injury arising from that occasion.

Not drinking alcohol is the safest option if you:

(8) drive or operate heavy machinery
(9) are pregnant, planning a pregnancy or breastfeeding
(10) are under 18 years of age.

Not drinking alcohol may also be the safest option if you:

(11) are taking other medications or drugs

116

(12) have a history of brain injury or liver disease.

Please check with your doctor if you are not sure.

AUDIT Score 16–19

Based on your responses, we recommend that you seek advice and support on how to reduce your drinking levels. Further information about risky drinking and the harms to your health can be found on the *SayWhen* website here. If you would like access to an alcohol and drug service in your local area, have a look at the help section at the bottom of the page.

How can I avoid risks from drinking?
To minimise your risk of harm from drinking, the National Health and Medical Research Council of Australia recommends the following guidelines:

For healthy men and women:

(13) drinking **no more than two standard drinks on any day** reduces the lifetime risk of harm from alcohol-related disease or injury
(14) drinking **no more than four standard drinks on a single occasion** reduces the risk of alcohol-related injury arising from that occasion.

Not drinking alcohol is the safest option if you:

(15) drive or operate heavy machinery
(16) are pregnant, planning a pregnancy or breastfeeding
(17) are under 18 years of age.

Not drinking alcohol may also be the safest option if you:

(18) are taking other medications or drugs
(19) have a history of brain injury or liver disease.

Please check with your doctor if you are not sure.

AUDIT Score 20+

Based on your responses, we strongly recommend that you speak to a specialist alcohol counselling service over the phone or online to discuss this further and to obtain referral for additional help. Further information about risky drinking and the harms to your health can be found on the *SayWhen* website here. If you would like access to an alcohol and drug service in your local area, have a look at the help section at the bottom of the page.

How can I avoid risks from drinking?
To minimise your risk of harm from drinking, the National Health and Medical Research Council of Australia recommends the following guidelines:

For healthy men and women:

(20) drinking **no more than two standard drinks on any day** reduces the lifetime risk of harm from alcohol-related disease or injury

(21) drinking **no more than four standard drinks on a single occasion** reduces the risk of alcohol-related injury arising from that occasion.

Not drinking alcohol is the safest option if you:

(22) drive or operate heavy machinery
(23) are pregnant, planning a pregnancy or breastfeeding
(24) are under 18 years of age.

Not drinking alcohol may also be the safest option if you:

(25) are taking other medications or drugs
(26) have a history of brain injury or liver disease.

Please check with your doctor if you are not sure.

DUDIT Score MALES: 1–5, FEMALES: 1

You may not need self-help advice, but if you are interested to know more about the effects of different drugs, we recommend the JustAskUs website and the information provided by the Australian Drug Foundation. If your substance use changes or you start to notice problems, you may like to repeat this screen to see if your risk has changed.

DUDIT Score MALES: 6–24, FEMALES: 2–24

You current substance use may be harmful to your health. You may find self-help advice useful – the JustAskUs website and the information provided by the Australian Drug Foundation might be helpful. We also recommend you speak to a specialist substance counsellor to find out more about your substance use and ways to manage any problems you are experiencing.

If you would like access to an alcohol and drug service in your local area, have a look at the help section at the bottom of the page.

DUDIT Score >24

We strongly recommended that you seek professional support to help you manage the problems you are experiencing with your substance use.

If you would like additional self-help advice, you may find the following websites useful: JustAskUs website and Australian Drug Foundation.

If you would like access to an alcohol and drug service in your local area, have a look at the help section at the bottom of the page.

GAMBLING

You may find the self-help advice on this site useful. There are also online and telephone support options that we recommend:

Gambling Help Online (www.gamblinghelponline.org.au)

Free 24 hour online support.

Also, you can further explore the impact of your gambling using this calculator: www. gamblinghelponline.org.au/regaining-control/gambling-calculator/

ASSIST

All drug use carries some level of risk – even medications can produce unwanted side effects. To find out more about each of the drugs you have used, please look at the information here. For some quick statistics on drug use in Australia, have a look at the information on the Australian Drug Foundation website.

It is important to remember that mixing drugs, especially with alcohol, can be unpredictable, dangerous and even fatal. This includes mixing alcohol with over-the-counter or prescribed medications. For example:

(1) **Alcohol + cannabis** may cause nausea, vomiting, panic, anxiety and paranoia.
(2) **Alcohol + energy drinks (with caffeine), ice, speed or ecstasy** may cause more risky behaviour, may place your body under great stress and may make an overdose more likely.
(3) **Alcohol + benzodiazepines** may increase the risk of becoming unconscious and stopping breathing.

To find out more about the risks of specific drugs and drug combinations, we recommend that you look at the information provided here and here.

Stem cell miracles or Russian roulette?: patients' use of digital media to campaign for access to clinically unproven treatments

Alan Petersen[a], Casimir MacGregor[a] and Megan Munsie[b]

[a]School of Social Sciences, Monash University, Victoria, Australia; [b]Stem Cells Australia, Department of Anatomy and Neuroscience, University of Melbourne, Victoria, Australia

In this article, we examine how patients use digital media to gain access to treatments that have yet to be clinically proven as safe and effective. Making reference to the case of an Australian patient who achieved notoriety following a *60 Minutes* television programme in 2014 following her travel to Russia to undertake stem cell treatment, in the article we discuss the dynamic interplay of discourses of hope, risk and trust in this digitally mediated context. As we argue, Web 2.0 digital media provides patient activists with a powerful means to generate their own framings of the significance of treatments especially when linked with more traditional media such as television. Our findings underline how citizens may use digital media to create 'communities of hope' that sustain optimistic portrayals of treatments that may be resistant to official, regulatory discourses of risk-benefit and trust. Patients' growing use of digital media, we conclude, necessitates a reconceptualisation of 'health' and 'risk' and approaches to regulating treatments that are unproven and hence deemed 'risky'.

Introduction

Digitalisation is profoundly shaping health care, including the operation of hospitals and other institutions and the practices of risk management and prevention. In this article, we draw on data from a project on so-called stem cell tourism (Petersen, Seear, & Munsie, 2014; Petersen, Tanner, & Munsie, 2015) to examine how patients may use digital media to gain access to clinically unproven – and hence potentially unsafe – treatments, namely stem cell treatments. Making reference to the plight of an Australian patient who travelled to Russia to undertake stem cell treatment and became a vocal patient activist for unproven stem cell treatments following a *60 Minutes* television programme in 2014, and extensive related media coverage and online discussion, we illustrate the dynamic interplay of contending discourses of hope, risk and trust that characterise the era of digitalised health and help to define the architecture of 'choice' that consumers of new treatments increasingly are compelled to navigate. As we argue, digital media has provided patient activists with a powerful tool for framing the significance of treatments, especially when they are linked with more traditional media such as television. In the article, we discuss the implications of this growing media-enabled activism – for how individuals conceptualise 'health' and 'risk', and for approaches to regulating treatments that are unproven and hence deemed 'risky'. To set the scene, we begin by outlining the broad context of digitalised health and its impacts, before turning to details of our study.

Digitalisation, health and risk

Digitalisation is profoundly shaping the practices and experiences of health, risk and health care (Lupton, 2013). The rise of the Internet and the change from Web 1.0's static webpages to Web 2.0's dynamic user-generated-content, involving social media like Facebook, Twitter and YouTube, has created new markets of health information, tests and treatments, and novel opportunities for 'consuming health' (Lupton, 2013; Mazanderani, O'Neill, & Powell, 2013; Murthy, 2012; Wen-Ying, Hunt, Folkers, & Augustson, 2011). Online journals or blogs, for example, enable citizens to share experiences of health and health care (such as weight loss) to offer mutual support for treatment endeavours and to bear witness to the benefits of self-care (Leggatt-Cook & Chamberlain, 2012). One of the most immediate, far reaching impacts of digitalisation has been on 'prosumption' – the production and consumption of digital content, whereby citizens can establish contact with and generate information for others who are physically remote and few in number (for example if suffering conditions that are rare), including patients, families, scientists and health professionals or treatment providers (including those based in other countries) (Ritzer & Jurgenson, 2010). Through Web 2.0, prosumers can create their own content, collaborate in fundraising, raise community awareness about particular conditions, and lobby for and contribute to research on promising treatments (Mazanderani et al., 2013; Murthy, 2012). In recent years, new patient forums and patient-led research endeavours, often involving collaborations with scientists, clinicians and health authorities, have emerged (Vayena, Brownsword, & Edwards et al., 2015). Digital media, especially social media networks, have enabled stories about new research or treatment breakthroughs or recovery to 'go viral' and thereby raise awareness and potentially heighten expectations of innovations. New digital technologies have also offered providers of treatments that are yet to be deemed by medical authorities and regulators to be effective and safe a new means of marketing their products, employing 'direct-to-consumer' advertising (Petersen & Seear, 2011) and their own social media platforms (Kamenova, Reshef, & Caulfield, 2014) to exploit the optimism surrounding new purportedly life-saving or life-enhancing treatments.

Writing more than two decades ago and well before the emergence of social media, Rabinow (1992) noted the then emergent forms of sociality based on biological identities, specifically associated with growing genetic diagnoses. Since then, others have documented the increasing significance of so-called biological citizenship based on shared biophysical characteristics (Petryna, 2002; Rose & Novas, 2005). Prosumer digital media content configures newer mutations of 'biosociality' and 'biological citizenship', with citizens playing an active role in building disease-specific patient communities that are oriented to realising particular hoped for futures by political, social and economic means. As Julien (2015) has argued, drawing on Bourdieu (1984), the interactions of digital inhabitants extend offline interactions, in that they involve conflict, exclusion and concealment, and efforts to achieve social distinction and build social capital. In their efforts to achieve social distinction, digital users create structures, rules and content that are unique to their communities (Julien, 2015, pp. 361–365).

The prosumption of digital media allows users to select and present information to gain some level of control over interactions and responses (Mazanderani et al., 2013). The concept of framing, widely used in media analysis, is useful in this context, in drawing attention to the ways in which digital users may give salience to certain information, values and perspectives, so as to invite particular interpretations and moral standpoints (Scheufele, 1999). By framing stories in certain ways, particularly during the early stages of an issue, event or innovation, digital users, like producers of older media, can limit the terms of a debate, about what exists, what happens, what matters and what demands attention (Gitlin, 1980; Miller & Riechert, 2000). In the case of new treatments, framing may include the use of certain language to describe different actors, such as patients, doctors and providers, along with the use of certain stories or story lines, and weblinks to information or images that invite certain interpretations of the significance of innovations. For example, there may be reference to only positive findings from research or photos of 'happy' patients receiving treatments, with little or no information on whether the actual improvement was transient or of a sustained and verified nature, or acknowledgement of any biophysical or financial risks encountered.

Patient-contributed forums, such as *PatientsLikeMe* and *CureTogether* and fund-raising ventures, such as *GoFundMe* and *PeoplePledge*, are pointing to novel modes of citizen interaction and identity creation that complement and, in some cases, supplant established interactions and identities. These forums have been made possible by digital media and would probably cease to exist without it. The limitations of traditional models of science communication and innovation, based on 'top-down', linear processes of knowledge production, transmission and translation, and relatively static content, have become evident with the advent of new media involving 'bottom-up', non-linear, distributed and multi-layered processes of communication and various social actors engaged in establishing and renegotiating the meanings of developments (Maeseele, Allgaier, & Martinelli, 2013). Citizens can create or jointly co-create and disseminate their own preferred narratives about themselves and their lives, about particular conditions and treatments and about those who provide and deny them, and become experts of their own conditions. Others, such as treatment providers, can also exploit new digital media platforms to promote their activities, by creating positive stories of treatments. These optimistic narratives, we suggest, are likely to play a crucial role in the 'political economy of hope' (DelVecchio Good, Good, Schaffer, & Lind, 1990) that underpins new and emerging treatment markets, especially when combined with other, more established forms of media such as television and print and online news media. The convergence of different digital media forms, with weblinks, blogs, Facebook and Twitter, for example, increasingly embedded within and linked to older media, ensures that stories of hope not only have potential short-term public impact but longer-term endurance (Murthy, 2012).

Some recent reported cases of citizen activism in relation to accessing treatments yet to be recognised by scientists and regulatory authorities as clinically proven (that is supported by evidence gathered in clinical trials) and therefore potentially unsafe and with unclear benefits, underline the significance of this new mediated environment for the political economy of hope. In one highly publicised case in Croatia in 2014, 'a subgroup of patients offered another group of patients [suffering the neurologic disease amyotrophic lateral sclerosis (ALS)] a financially covered "package" for a [stem cell] treatment in a hospital in China without consulting their doctors or other Croatian medical experts' (Mitrečić, Bilić, & Gajović, 2014). It was reported that a number of Croatian celebrities were involved in an 'ice-bucket challenge', whereby someone dumped a bucket of ice water on someone's head, to help raise funds for the amyotrophic lateral sclerosis patients and that several patient organisations had appeared in prime time shows which talked about this 'strange disease for which the only hope exists in stem cells clinics in Asia' (Mitrečić et al., 2014, p. 443). The 'ice-bucket challenge' event was the subject of 'a number of newspaper articles and TV broadcasts', and went viral on social media, particularly in the USA, during July–August, 2014, where a similar event was held. In the aftermath of the challenge, Facebook estimated that '28 million people posted about ALS between June 1 and August 28, including comments and tags. 2.4 million videos also were created on YouTube, spreading the word like wildfire' (Goulart, 2014). The event was deemed by media and communication specialists to be a marketing success by embracing 'the community spirit of social media', and providing 'the low barrier to entry means everyone can get involved and feel as though they've done something good with their day' (Adeyeri, 2014). The event was also clearly a fundraising success with more than $22 million received in donations, ten times more than the same time period for the previous year (ALS Association, 2015).

The amyotrophic lateral sclerosis case highlighted how citizens, aided by digital media, may quickly mobilise to build optimism in communities, to raise often-substantial funds to support research and to help citizens gain access to treatments otherwise unavailable to them, and in the process bypass accredited experts and perceived regulatory or bureaucratic hurdles. The Australian case that we analyse further demonstrates the power of digital media, especially how social media may link with and gain leverage from more established media to create 'communities of hope' that may run counter to official discourses of risk-benefit and trust. It involved a patient, Kristy Cruise, whose plight became a *cause célèbre* following a *60 Minutes* television programme on her journey to Russia to receive stem cell treatments.

Method

The case of Kristy Cruise, namely the coverage of her story on *60 Minutes* and subsequent news reports and social media communication concerning her plight, achieved prominence during the course of our study of so-called stem cell tourism (Petersen et al., 2014; Petersen et al., 2015). It is one of a number of cases that came to our attention where individual patients had achieved a media profile following their efforts to gain access to stem cell treatments that are unproven and hence deemed 'risky'. The case offered the opportunity to explore how patient activists use digital media and gain leverage from their media profile to draw attention to their plight and to the benefits of stem cell treatments. Consequently, we sought to explore Cruise's use of digital media in the context of and in relation to wider media communication on the case.

Media and internet content relating to the Kirsty Cruise were searched on the Internet using a combination of keywords, such as 'Kirsty Cruise, 'MS', and '60 minutes'. Data was restricted to Australian content only that appeared between January 2014 and July 2015 ($n = 169$). A range of media content was collected including television news stories, interviews, print news stories, blog posts and social media posts. Interview and collected media content were inductively coded using thematic analysis utilising Gibbs' (2007) framework which included: familiarisation and immersion in data, code building, conformity and discrepancy within theme development, and data consolidation and interpretation.

Our analytical approach was informed by critical discourse analysis to help us uncover the implicit and taken-for-granted values, assumptions and origins of seemingly neutral, self-evident media content, and how they relate to dominant ideologies and power in discourses (Van Dijk, 2005). Critical discourse analysis allows one insight into the social production of texts and adds a linguistic approach to understanding the relationship between language and practice, and focuses on the way in which theories of 'reality' and relations of power are encoded in such aspects of syntax, style, rhetorical devices and semiotics within media texts (Lupton, 1992). We gained ethical approval for the project through Monash University's human research ethics committee (CF12/1532 201000832).

Findings: competing discourses of hope and risk

Stem cell treatments, like other experimental treatments (for example for cancer) that are yet to be clinically proven, are the subject of competing discourses of hope and risk and, often trust. On the one hand, discourses of hope pervade patients' and carers' narratives regarding treatment decisions and the online advertising materials of providers who aim to profit from 'capitalising hope' (Martin, Brown, & Turner, 2008). On the other, regulators, scientists and medical authorities promulgate precautionary, risk-benefit discourses, in regard to treatments offered by those who reside at the margins of medicine (see International Society for Stem Cell Research [ISSCR], 2015; National Health and Medical Research Council [NHMRC], 2015; Stem Cells Australia [SCA], 2015). These strongly pro-science advisors often draw a distinction between 'realistic hope' based on feasible, evidence-based intervention scenarios and 'false hope', seen as based on no credible evidence and hence 'risky' (Petersen et al., 2014; Petersen et al., 2015).

Discourses of hope circulate widely on the Internet, increasingly via the numerous online patient forums and social media platforms that have emerged in recent years, and coexist and compete with contending discourses of risk and risk-benefit, created and disseminated largely by scientists, clinicians, bioethicists and regulatory authorities. The Internet has been found to be an important source of information for prospective patients, while social media are increasingly used to gain information about health and risk, to share experiences about treatments, to track others' health experiences, to monitor one's own weight, diet or other health indicators or symptoms, and to raise money for or draw attention to a health-related issues (Fox, 2011, pp. 2–3).

Facebook dominates the social media space and in recent years the level of user engagement with the platform has increased markedly. A survey undertaken in September 2014 found that more than 50% of online adults use two or more social media platforms, a significant increase from 2013, with Facebook being the most popular platform (Duggan, Ellison, Lampe, Lenhart, & Madden, 2015). Social media, we suggest, offers patients a significant means for forging communities of hope and disseminating optimistic narratives about particular treatments and providers; further, these narratives tend to run counter to official rational discourses focusing on probabilistic assessments of personal harms and precautionary practices.

However, the potential of social media to heighten such optimism is magnified when they are linked to more established media such as newspapers and television. The rise of the Internet and social media has vastly extended the capacity for this more established media to reach out to and engage with audiences in ways that potentially shape responses to new experimental treatments, including constructions of risk. Digitalisation allows the creation of stories over time, which may linger on websites and other media long after a story has played out off screen or offline and create a particular skewed portrayal of issues and events, leading audiences with little understanding of alternative perspectives, in this case regulator's warnings about the risks posed by treatments.

Kristy Cruise gained prominence following the screening of the programme, 'Russian Roulette: the radical procedure that could change lives', which appeared on Channel 9's *60 Minutes* on 9 March 2014. It covered Cruise's journey to Russia to receive stem cell treatment for her MS and discussed at some length an Australian hospital's 'decision to discontinue stem cell treatment for MS patients'. *60 Minutes*, which has been shown in prime time on Sunday evenings continually since 1979, is a version of the much longer running USA newsmagazine programme by the same name. In recent years, the pro-gramme has consistently ranked in the top 15 (and at times within the top 5) Australian television programmes with an audience of at least 1.5 million (OZTam, 2015), and the issues covered and the individuals who are featured often achieve considerable promi-nence, especially with the rise of social media. One can find past episodes of the programme on YouTube, and the programme has a Twitter account and Facebook page, thus ensuring stories' endurance and wide distribution.

In framing 'Russian Roulette', *60 Minutes* positioned itself as highly sympathetic to the plight of Cruise and as an ally in her quest to receive treatment. Australian hospitals and regulatory authorities, on the other hand, were posited as uncaring and out of touch. Scientists' and regulatory agencies' warnings about the risks of unproven stem cell treatments (ISSCR, 2015; NHMRC, 2015; SCA, 2015) were largely ignored. Like some earlier cases involving patients' or carers' pursuit of treatments that fall foul of regulations that have been taken up by the media (e.g. Petersen, Anderson, & Allan, 2005), *60 Minutes* adopted an advocacy role, highlighting the 'injustices' encountered by families in their quest to obtain 'saviour' treatments and the culpability of the uncaring authorities who denied them access to them.

Cruise's story, which included a strong character, a clear plot, tragedy, conflict, suspension and eventual resolution via a successful outcome, was bound to attract media and public attention. Cruise is a young, 'happily married' mother from what is portrayed as an ordinary family that is struck by the tragedy of illness and 'forced' (a term used repeatedly by the reporter in 'Russian Roulette') to seek treatment overseas, thus submitting herself to financial and physical risks and the emotional pain associated with having to travel and leave her family and support for the unknown. Being a nurse by profession, it was implied that she is especially well placed to undertake effective research and make a valid judgement on treatments.

In the story, Cruise is portrayed as a 'warrior' – and indeed describes herself as a 'HSCT (Hematopoietic Stem Cell Transplant) Warrior' on her Twitter page – who, like a number of other high-profile patient-advocates of unproven stem cell treatments, such as the Australians Perry Cross and footballer Adam Goodes, and more recently the American ice hockey legend Gordon 'Gordie' Howe and his family – have achieved a considerable profile via media appearances in their quest to pursue treatments. These latter individuals were already celebrities, and all struck by the misfortune of illness or injury and all positioned and/or positioning themselves as vanguards in the 'movement' to gain access to a new promising treatment. Their tragedy and profile, and heroic struggles, have combined to bring public attention to and provide a particular framing of an issue, as celebrities have for other issues (Anderson, Petersen, Wilkinson, & Allan, 2009). While Cruise did not have the same profile to begin with, her story soon gave her a profile that attracted considerable public attention. Her plight as an ordinary mother confronted with tragedy invited understandable sympathy.

'Russian Roulette' opens with a teary Cruise, who comments, 'My kids are young – accepting it [the condition] is not an option', and then follows her as she prepares to travel to Russia, including having her head shaved in readiness for her treatment (presented as a kind of ritual degradation ceremony), wishing her children and husband farewell, under-taking the treatment, and her 'miraculous' recovery 6 months following her return. Cruise is depicted as a strong-willed heroic figure fighting for justice, namely the treatment that is denied her at home, and, as explained via a voiceover accompanying a picture of Cruise in a hospital bed in Russia, 'will swap the comforts of home in Queensland for a grueling round of chemotherapy and stem cell treatment in a Russian hospital'. As she heads off, the reporter comments: 'A long and expensive journey into the unknown and all on her own. It will be close to $100,000, but watching Kristy shake uncontrollably perhaps not a moment too soon.'

In our research on stem cell tourism we found that patients often express frustration with not having access to stem cell treatments in Australia and often depicted doctors as being indifferent or unhelpful (Petersen et al., 2014). Cruise, too, is portrayed as being denied a potentially life-saving treatment in Australia: 'To treat multiple sclerosis in this way is groundbreaking and the results can be extraordinary. But Kristy has been forced to come here [Russia] because in Australia treatment has been deemed by health bureaucrats as experimental.' The implication is that treatments would be safe or safer if offered in Australia. However, Cruise's decision to travel abroad for treatment, and to refuse conventional drug treatment, is portrayed not as reckless bravado and undue concern for risk, as might be suggested by the programmes's title, 'Russian Roulette', but rather well researched and considered. When asked by the interviewer, 'Do you feel that by going to Russia you are playing Russian roulette?', she responds in an unequivocal manner: 'No. I have made a very careful decision. I don't think it is Russian roulette at all.'

In the programme, the drama of her story is reinforced by the appearance of a would-be-saviour Australian doctor who is thwarted in its attempts to assist Cruise. The doctor, Collin Andrews, who previously worked at Canberra Hospital, is described as 'one of the few neurologists in Australia willing to carry out the stem cell treatment that could change Kristy's life, but he isn't allowed to'. In an interview segment, the doctor underlines the effectiveness and relative safety of the procedure, responding to a question about how successful the treatment is: 'In most cases, it stops the disease in its tracks; there are no further relapses; no presence of the disease'. Further, to underline its safety, he employs a risk–benefit analysis to justify patients' decisions:

> In the early days it had a mortality rate of nine percent, just over a decade ago, but now it's down to less than one percent. And, given that some people will die from their disease and be severely disabled or maybe in a nursing home, the patients are much freer about taking the risks than the doctors are.

In this portrayal, the risk, namely death or disability, is portrayed as small and borne by patients who are less constrained ('freer') than doctors 'about taking the risks' because, it is implied, there is more at stake ('some people will die…and be disabled or maybe in a nursing home'). This low-risk yet high potential benefit narrative is reinforced by the 'saviour' doctor in Russia, who comments that he has had an 'eighty percent success' and has had 'no deaths in eight years of treating MS patients'. He also recounted his success in treating one patient who is no longer wheel-chair-bound.

Cruise's story has the characteristic happy ending, in this case a 'miraculous' recovery. In the final shots, she is shown running along a beach with her husband and, when interviewed, comments, 'It just feels like me again'. A voiceover observes: 'For MS patients like Kristy and Lauren [another patient "denied" treatment in Australia and who appears on the programme] and their families, the greatest reward will be if more Australian doctors just look at the evidence and get the message.' In response to a question about the medical proof that her MS has 'halted in some way', Cruise responds that her neurologist has told her that she has 'less lesions now and the ones that are there are smaller' and that 'that's a miracle because they never said they would take away lesions.' Cruise recounts feeling 'really sad' that other patients aren't able to access stem cell treatments and fortunate in having the resources and knowledge and 'shear willpower' to get to Russia, and that 'it just seems like madness that we can't do this in Australia. It breaks my heart. It really breaks my heart.'

The screening of 'Russian Roulette' was not the end of Cruises' story. In its aftermath, *60 Minutes* website created links to Cruise's blog and website, and posted the web address of the clinic in Moscow that she visited and that of another 'pioneer of stem cell treatment for MS' and a statement from the Australian hospital which was mentioned in the programme as terminating its schedule of stem cell treatments, along with questions posed by *60 Minutes* (noted as being 'still unanswered or entirely ignored'). *60 Minutes'* website also included a link to a short video with a reflection by the interviewer describing her puzzlement in regards to the Australian hospital's decision to discontinue stem cell treatment for MS, and 'links to some of the latest research'. These digital links have contributed to the story's endurance and potential impact. Although there is no way of gauging the overall response of audiences to the programme, postings on *60 Minutes* Facebook page after the showing of 'Russian Roulette' were mostly supportive of its moral stance: for example, 'WHY don't we undertake this procedure in Australia for MSer's that want to put THEIR own bodies on the line and try. Please anybody that believes in fairness and in lending a helping hand: PLEASE SHARE THIS POST'. On one of *60 Minutes* websites, posted in May 2014, it is noted that 'the response [to Cruise's story] was simply extraordinary' and that 'for the thousands of Australian MS patients, Kristy's story is an inspiration.' In short, both 'Russian Roulette's' account of the issues, and *60 Minutes'* subsequent homepage postings and weblinks served to create a lasting optimistic portrayal of stem cell treatments and of the plight of those seeking them.

This portrayal is assisted through the omission of certain perspectives and information – significantly, as noted, regulators' concerns and warnings about the risks of unproven stem cell treatments outlined in various publications and websites, including patient information sources, such as those referred to. During the programme, only *one* qualification regarding stem cell treatments is offered: 'It's important to emphasize the treatment doesn't work for everyone with MS. You need to be young, preferably under age 40 and in the early stages of the disease; Kristy Cruise should be the ideal candidate, but under Australian protocols she is not eligible because she hasn't tried and failed conventional drug treatments.' Furthermore, there is no response to the Australian hospital's media statement indicating 'limited research data on the efficacy and outcomes of this treatment from studies undertaken to date', the potential for 'more risks than long term benefits' for most patients of MS from this treatment, and outlining its processes for referring more complex cases to another Australian hospital which offers a programme with 'strict eligibility criteria' for stem cell transplant for patients with MS.

Hope trumps risk?

Cruise, like some other patient advocates, has proved adept at using digital media, namely Facebook, to capitalise on the profile her *60 Minutes* appearance has given her to create a strong online presence and a 'community of hope', comprising fellow patients, their families and supporters. In September 2015, her homepage registered '4,781 Likes'. In another Australian television programme, SBS *Insight*, also screened in 2014 and in which Cruise appeared and which also focused strongly on patients' endeavours to gain treatments, she claimed to have responded to '37,000 emails in four months' and to have a further 12,000 emails in her account that she had not responded to. New digital media, when allied with older media, has provided patients like Cruise with a significant platform to voice their views, to put forward positive views about treatments and to contribute to a discourse of hope that runs counter to the risk and risk–benefit discourses promulgated by scientists, regulators and other pro-science groups.

Titled 'Moving mountains to defeat MS', Cruise's webpage, which had its first post a year before 'Russian Roulette' (March 9, 2014), offers a kind of 'drop-in centre' or 'one-stop-shop' for those wishing to learn about MS and stem cell treatments and providers, and offers an optimistic depiction of what treatments can deliver. The Facebook page includes almost-daily blogs by Cruise; links to various publications, guidelines, and 'carers' information for Moscow'; recommendations on certain providers; photos, many of Cruise alone or with others, and some with inspirational quotes (for example 'when confronted with a stranger's unimaginable pain, CHOOSE courage', 'dreams don't work unless you do'); videos, some of Cruise in Russia, one featuring Cruise drawing a raffle for a sun screen product and another her promoting the same product ('particularly applicable for people with MS'); and stories about and correspondence from other patients, from providers and from Cruise herself offering advice and encouraging patients to undertake their own research. For example, in one post, she comments,

> I can verify that all facilities listed are reputable hospitals, with haematologists overseeing the transplants. I have personally spoken to at least one patient who has been to every facility on the list. I have also spoken to many of the doctors. There are no scam clinics here. No scam doctors. And all offer genuine HSCT [Hematopoietic Stem Cell Transplant].

She also warns about what she considers to be dubious stem cell therapy being offered in Australia and that she is 'sick of hearing sad stories from people who have fallen for this scam and lost $10,000+...'.

What is important to note about the posts on Cruises' Facebook page, that is common to other prosumer sites, is that the owner has the power to frame the issues, such as risk; to create a narrative through time that goes beyond the individual postings. Thus, individual postings are not always treatment related, with some focusing on daily events and interesting items of information, employing various media; for example YouTube clips. Such postings serve to show visitors that Cruise has a non-patient identity and is 'just like them', thus engendering empathy, trust, and a sense of camaraderie and community among followers.

Visitors to Cruise's Facebook page do not know how information has been 'doctored' – to use a phrase of one of the respondents in our study when commenting on her webpage – and the page includes no information on risks and warnings found in expert sources, noted earlier. In one post, Cruise has sought to 'correct' what she sees as another poster's misrepresentation of the efficacy of stem cell treatment following a television news story of an Australian with MS travelling abroad for stem cell treatment. The poster commented, 'I was following a guy who went through this treatment in Russia & he has stopped posting, which I think means it hasn't worked?' Cruise soon replied: 'I have not heard of a single person who went to Moscow from Australia who has said it didn't work. Most patients tend to stop blogging when they get back because they are initially recovering from the chemo'.

Some weeks later, Cruise posted an 'HSCT Patient List (Australia)', with Cruise listed as the first patient to have 'completed treatment', in 2013, and a list of 30 patients in 2014 to have 'completed treatment', 59 listed for 2015 at various stages of treatment, and others listed for treatments in 2016 and 2017 – offering in effect an endorsement of treatments for others who may be contemplating travelling. On 4 August, 2014, *Multiple Sclerosis News Today*, a disease-specific news website, posted a message, noting that Australian authorities were alerting MS patients to the risks posed by unproven stem cell treatments offered in Australian and overseas following the death of an Australian woman in Russia (Farreira, 2014).

Discussion

Patients' growing use of digital media – including to lobby for and to gain access to treatments that are unproven and hence deemed 'risky' – should encourage scholars to reflect on how they conceive 'health' and 'risk' and their relationship. Over a period of nearly 50 years, the social sciences have produced a rich body of theory on how risks are constructed, communicated and politicised, including in the contexts of health, medicine and health care. In her seminal text, *Purity and Danger* (1966), Douglas, for example, explored how objective risks are transformed into social risks for a group that needed to be managed. More recently, Castel (1991) documented the rise of new 'preventive strategies of social administration' that replaced the notion of the subject, who is controlled directly by others (for example carers, experts) via face-to-face encounters, with 'the factors of risk' involving abstract calculations of risk and related surveillance and technologies of administration. The recent rapid development and adoption of digital media, such as social media, however, necessitates a substantial reconceptualisation of 'health' and 'risk' and their relationship. Increasingly, citizens are using digital media to actively manage and redefine their own health and risk, by seeking expert advice, products and services online and by producing and sharing knowledge that may sometimes run counter to established expert discourses (Petersen, 2015, pp. 88–93). They are becoming experts of their own conditions and sometimes challenging official definitions of risk and risk-benefit. As we argued, prosumption is profoundly changing the meanings and practices of health, medicine and health care – as seen in the case of Kristy Cruise.

Before the rise of Web 2.0 media, Cruise's story may have attracted short-term public interest, but may not have endured as a focal point for patient activism, unless the individual had the high profile needed to attracted funds to support a campaign. In the stem cell field, Christopher Reeve's effort to advance stem cell research is the most prominent example. However, social media has enabled ordinary citizen-patients with a much lower profile to achieve prominence, using social media, to highlight their plight, to create and market a unique identity, and to disseminate optimistic narratives about treatments, sometimes for self-promotional purposes. The creation of narratives in real-time enabled via social media provides such stories with an immediacy and a degree of personalisation and audience connection that finds no parallel with traditional media, such as television.

New digital media provides a powerful platform for constructing and communicating risk, especially for citizen-patients who are able to create narratives about themselves and their own lives, including the 'truth' regarding the efficacy and safety of particular treatments and the trustworthiness of providers. As we have argued, drawing on data from a study on stem cell tourism which included the case of Kristy Cruise who undertook stem cell treatment in Russia, Web 2.0 user-generated-content social media provides a significant means for citizens to build and lead biosocial 'communities of hope' that create optimistic 'framings' of particular treatments and conceptions of risk. With the growing emphasis on self-care and patient expertise, citizens – especially those who have achieved public prominence via other media, such as Cruise – are well placed to frame issues in ways that resonate with their audiences who, in many cases, are patients with conditions that are otherwise untreatable. As argued, digitalisation enables patient stories, such as those of technological optimism (Petersen & Seear, 2011), to be stored and circulated long after events have played out off screen or offline, giving them potential impact over time. This makes these stories a key element in the reconfiguring of risk and sustaining a political economy of hope; in countering alternative claims about the benefits and risks of treatments and the trustworthiness of providers. Stories may be framed in ways that enable prosumers to construct discourses of risk that may differ from expert discourses.

Conclusion

The growing use of digital media by patients to create communities of hope that campaign for access to unproven treatments should lead regulators to reflect on the implications and limitations of their own approaches to 'regulating risk'. These approaches generally employ 'top-down', relatively static forms of communication and a precautionary, risk-oriented rationality often based on abstract principles (such as 'do no harm', 'respect for autonomy') that pays insufficient attention to the novel forms of sociability and communication that have arisen with digital health. Our own data and recent evidence on patient activism referred to in the article highlight emergent patient communities that may be largely impervious to conventional regulatory approaches to risk, since they are bound by strong affective sentiments of hope. Unlike the static content of Web 1.0, the prosumption of Web 2.0 media provides ordinary citizens with the capacity to constantly recreate and rapidly disseminate information, share experiences, and challenge officially authorised stories, including the risk-focused, precautionary accounts of scientists, regulators, and other authorities. As noted, Facebook is a place where users may share criticisms of doctors and of what they see as uncaring authorities. It is in such communities, we contend, that hope tends to trump expert constructions of risk and risk-benefit and that undertaking treatment is seen to be, as some of our patients reasoned, 'worth the risk', or to involve risks that were deemed to be 'small'.

In understanding the role activists play within new treatment markets, and in particular how they use digital media to build communities of hope and create optimistic narratives that mitigate risk, regulators will be better placed to develop strategies that respond to the conditions of digitalised health, including the means for engaging with citizens that are more imaginative and personally meaningful.

Disclosure statement

No potential conflict of interest was reported by the authors.

Funding

This work was supported by the Australian Research Council [grant number DP120100921];

References

Adeyeri, A. (2014, August 27). Ice bucket challenge: What are the lessons for marketers. *The Guardian*. Retrieved September 2, 2015, from http://www.theguardian.com/media-network/media-network-blog/2014/aug/27/ice-bucket-challenge-lessons-marketing
ALS Association. (2015). Ice bucket challenge donations reach $22.9 million to the ALS Association. *News release*. August 19, 2014. Retrieved September 2, 2015, from http://www.alsa.org/news/media/press-releases/ice-bucket-challenge-081914.html

Anderson, A., Petersen, A., Wilkinson, C., & Allan, S. (2009). *Nanotechnology, risk and commu-nication*. Houndmills: Palgrave Macmillan.

Bourdieu, P. (1984). *Distinction: A social critique of the judgement of taste*. Cambridge, MA: Harvard University Press.

Castel, R. (1991). From dangerousness to risk. In G. Burchell, C. Gordon, & P. Miller (Eds.), *The Foucault effect: Studies in governmentality* (pp. 281–298). London: Harvester Wheatsheaff.

Cruise, K. (2014). Moving mountains to defeat MS. *Facebook page*. Retrieved May 11, 2015, from https://www.facebook.com/MovingMountainsForKristy

DelVecchio Good, M.-J., Good, B. J., Schaffer, C., & Lind, S. E. (1990). American oncology and the discourse on hope. *Culture, Medicine and Psychiatry, 14*, 59–79. doi:10.1007/BF00046704

Douglas, M. (1966). *Purity and danger: An analysis of the concepts of pollution and taboo*. London: Ark Paperbacks.

Duggan, M., Ellison, N. B., Lampe, C., Lenhart, A., & Madden, M. (2015, April 10). Social media update 2014. *Pew Research Centre, Internet, Science and Tech*. Retrieved from http://www. pewinternet.org/2015/01/09/social-media-update-2014/

Farreira, L. M. (2014). Update: Australian authorities warn about unapproved MS stem cell treatments after death in Russia. *Multiple Sclerosis News Today*. Retrieved May 11, 2015, from http://multiplesclerosisnewstoday.com/2014/08/04/update-australian-authorities-warn-about-unapproved-ms-stem-cell-treatments-after-death-in-russia/

Fox, S. (2011). *The social life of health information, 2011*.Washington, DC: Pew Research Centre's Internet and American Life Project. Retrieved April 13, 2015, from http://www.pewinternet.org/ files/old-media/Files/Reports/2011/PIP_Social_Life_of_Health_Info.pdf

Gibbs, G. (2007). *Analyzing qualitative data*. London: Sage.

Gitlin, T. (1980). *The whole world is watching: Mass media in the making and unmaking of the new Left*. Berkeley, CA: University of California Press.

Goulart, J. (2014, December 18). The data behind the ALS ice bucket challenge. *IBM Big Data & Analytics Hub*. Retrieved September 2, 2015, from http://www.ibmbigdatahub.com/blog/data-behind-als-ice-bucket-challenge

ISSCR: International Society for Stem Cell Research. (2015). Frequently asked questions. Retrieved May 12, 2015, from http://www.isscr.org/visitor-types/public/stem-cell-faq

Julien, C. (2015). Bourdieu, social capital and online interaction. *Sociology, 49*(2), 356–373. doi:10.1177/0038038514535862

Kamenova, K., Reshef, A., & Caulfield, T. (2014). Representations of stem cell clinics on Twitter. *Stem Cell Reviews and Reports, 10*, 753–760. doi:10.1007/s12015-014-9534-z

Leggatt-Cook, C., & Chamberlain, K. (2012). Blogging for weight loss: Personal accountability, writing selves, and the weight-loss blogosphere. *Sociology of Health & Illness, 34*(7), 963–977. doi:10.1111/shil.2012.34.issue-7

Lupton, D. (1992). Discourse analysis: A new methodology for understanding the ideologies of health and illness. *Australian Journal of Public Health, 16*(2), 145–150. doi:10.1111/j.1753-6405.1992.tb00043.x

Lupton, D. (2013). The digitally engaged patient: Self-monitoring and self-care in the digital health era. *Social Theory & Health, 11*, 256–270. doi:10.1057/sth.2013.10

Maeseele, P., Allgaier, J., & Martinelli, L. (2013). Bio-objects and the media: The role of commu-nication in bio-objectification processes. *Croatian Medical Journal, 54*(3), 301–305. doi:10.3325/cmj.2013.54.301

Martin, P., Brown, N., & Turner, A. (2008). Capitalizing hope: The commercial development of umbilical cord blood stem cell banking. *New Genetics and Society, 27*(2), 127–143. doi:10.1080/14636770802077074

Mazanderani, F., O'Neill, B., & Powell, J. (2013). "People power" or "pester power"? YouTube as a forum for the generation of evidence and patient advocacy. *Patient Education and Counseling, 93*(3), 420–425. doi:10.1016/j.pec.2013.06.006

Miller, M., & Riechert, B. P. (2000). Interest group strategies and journalistic norms: News media framing of environmental issues. In S. Allan, B. Adam, & C. Carter (Eds.), *Environmental risks and the media*. London: Routledge.

Mitrečić, D., Bilić, E., & Gajović, S. (2014). How Croatian patients suffering from amyotrophic lateral sclerosis have been turned into medical tourists – a comment on a medical and social phenomenon. *Croatian Medical Journal, 55*, 443–445. doi:10.3325/cmj.2014.55.443

Murthy, D. (2012). *Twitter: Social communication in the Twitter age*. Cambridge: Polity Press.

NHMRC: National Health and Medical Research Council. (2015). Stem Cell Treatments. Retrieved May 12, 2015, from https://www.nhmrc.gov.au/health-topics/stem-cell-treatments

OZTam. (2015). 'Search result' for *60-Minutes*. Retrieved April 13, 2015, from http://www.oztam. com.au/SearchResults.aspx?q=60%20minutes

Petersen, A. (2015). *Hope in health: The socio-politics of optimism*. Basingstoke: Palgrave Macmillan.

Petersen, A., Anderson, A., & Allan, S. (2005). Science fiction/science fact: Medical genetics in news stories. *New Genetics and Society, 24*(3), 337–353. doi:10.1080/14636770500350088

Petersen, A., & Seear, K. (2011). Technologies of hope: Techniques of the online advertising of stem cell treatments. *New Genetics and Society, 30*(4), 329–346. doi:10.1080/14636778.2011.592003

Petersen, A., Seear, K., & Munsie, M. (2014). Therapeutic journeys: The hopeful travails of stem cell tourists. *Sociology of Health & Illness, 36*(5), 670–685. doi:10.1111/shil.2014.36.issue-5

Petersen, A., Tanner, C., & Munsie, M. (2015). Between hope and evidence: How community advisors demarcate the boundary between legitimate and illegitimate stem cell treatments. *Health, 19*(2), 188–206.

Petryna, A. (2002). *Life exposed: Biological citizens after Chernobyl*. Princeton, NJ: Princeton University Press.

Rabinow, P. (1992). Artificiality and enlightenment: From sociobiology to biosociality. In J. Crary & S. Kwinter (Eds.), *Incorporations*. New York, NY: Urzone.

Ritzer, G., & Jurgenson, N. (2010). Production, consumption, prosumption: The nature of capitalism in the age of the digital prosumer. *Journal of Consumer Culture, 10*(1), 13–36. doi:10.1177/1469540509354673

Rose, N., & Novas, C. (2005). Biological citizenship. In A. Ong & S. J. Collier (Eds.), *Global assemblages: Technology, politics and ethics as anthropological problems*. London: Blackwell.

SCA: Stem Cells Australia. (2015). Patient information. Retrieved May 11, 2015. from http://www.stemcellsaustralia.edu.au/AboutUs/Document-Library/Patient-Information.aspx

Scheufele, D. A. (1999). Framing as a theory of media effects. *Journal of Communication, 49*(1), 103–122. doi:10.1111/jcom.1999.49.issue-1

Van Dijk, T. (2005). Critical discourse analysis. In D. Schiffrin, D. Tannen, & H. Hamilton (Eds.), *The handbook of discourse analysis* (pp. 352–371). Malden, MA: Blackwell Publishers Ltd. doi:10.1002/9780470753460.ch18

Vayena, E., Brownsword, R., Edwards, S. J., Greshake, B., Kahn, J. F., Ladher, N., … Tasioulas, J. (2015). Research led by participants: A new social contract for a new kind of research. *Journal of Medical Ethics*, Published online first April 13. doi:10.1136/medethics-2015-102663

Wen-Ying, S., Hunt, Y., Folkers, A., & Augustson, E. (2011). Cancer survivorship in the age of YouTube and social media: A narrative analysis. *Journal of Medical Internet Research, 13*(1), e–7. doi:10.2196/jmir.1569

Biosensing: how citizens' views illuminate emerging health and social risks

Maggie Mort, Celia Mary Roberts, Mette Kragh Furbo, Joann Wilkinson
and Adrian Mackenzie

Department of Sociology, Lancaster University, Lancaster, UK

This article explores material from a citizen's inquiry into the social and ethical implications of health biosensors. In 'Our Bodies, Our Data' a space was afforded for members of the public to examine two forms of health biosensing, and for the authors to research what happens when such examination shifts from the domain of experts to that of citizens. Drawing on data from this inquiry, which form part of a wider research project, 'Living Data: making sense of health biosensors', we open up conceptual and methodological questions about how to study innovative health technologies and contribute to debates about the direction of health biosensing by bringing forward the views of a group rarely heard in this domain: the public. The panel of 15 participants was shown examples, handled devices and heard evidence about the development of home ovulation monitoring and direct-to-consumer genetic testing. Citizens identified key areas of concern around the development, design and marketing of these devices, implicating technology companies, public bodies and civil society organisations. The panel articulated serious concerns relating to ethics, trust, accountability, quality and governance of health biosensors that operate 'outside the clinic'. Their deliberations reflect concern for what kind of society is being made when genetic testing and home reproductive technologies are promoted and sold directly to the public. The panel process allowed us to re-imagine biosensors, wresting their narratives from the individualising discourses of self-optimisation and responsibilisation which have dominated their introduction in Euro-US markets.

Introduction

Monitoring one's physiological state through the collection of personal bodily data – heart rate, temperature, sleep cycles, calories consumed, steps walked – is an increasingly important element of many people's attempts to achieve health and avoid risks of illness and medical intervention (Lupton, 2015). Self-monitoring promises to reduce and manage risk, but does it also produce new risks for individuals and for society?

Devices used in personal health monitoring practices are often referred to as 'biosensors' (Nafus, 2013). This contemporary term blends two entities: *devices* and *biologically active* agents (OED, 2011): implied in 'device' is the idea of collection, recording and storing or 'data-fying' what is being sensed from the *bio* (in the cases we describe here, saliva). Adding this process of data-fying to the commercial, 'direct-to-consumer' (DTC) context of

133

biosensing devices and practices, raises serious political, ethical and social concerns. Most research in this field, however, studies 'users' of self-tracking technologies and/or focuses on the technologies as 'kit'. Focusing on two key areas of health risk – in/fertility and dementia – in this article, we, in contrast, explore what citizens have to say about the risks and promises of biosensing.

'Lay' interpretation of risk and biosensors

Biosensors are iconic examples of the contemporary materialisation of risk. Building on the growing body of ethnographically informed work on information-based enhancement and augmentation of the body (such as Viseu & Suchman, 2010), in this article we add a public perspective on the development, use and implications of health monitoring devices 'outside the clinic'. The citizens' views reported here give an empirical perspective to sociological critiques of risk and rationality, articulating ways in which the decisions of so-called consumers of health biosensors are deeply embedded in complex lived realities of ontological insecurity and erosion of trust in professional and expert knowledges and services.

The ethnographically informed scenario used in our citizen's panel discussions (which we discuss more fully in the Methodology section) articulate two main forms of health risk: knowing one's future risk of dementia (driven in this case by anxiety and family circumstances); and warding off the risk of infertility and the physically and emotionally challenging medical interventions now commonly associated with it. The characters in our scenario engaging with these forms of medicalising risk have a sense of themselves as about to become pathologised and of needing to consider and address their health futures.

Managing future health risk through attention and action in the present is a strong theme in contemporary health discourses and is documented in studies of genetic testing, heart disease, fertility and HIV/AIDS. Much of this research, however, shows that in contrast to expert, statistical discourses, 'lay' people interpret future health risks in relational terms: thinking about family, personal connections and the authenticity of the source of knowledge. Roberts and Franklin (2004), for example show that couples at high risk of passing on serious genetic disease consider multiple factors (personal, familial and societal) in their decision-making about how to manage the risks of having a(nother) child with the condition. Similarly, in a study of ovarian cancer, Hallowell suggests that:

> [R]isk awareness is, at least in part, dependent upon the recognition of suffering in oneself and others, while managing risk is, among other things, an attempt to avoid suffering in the future for oneself and other family members. (Hallowell, 2006 p. 23)

In relation to the management of risk associated with the introduction of remote (sensor based) home care monitoring for older people, or 'telecare', it has been noted that there is also a shift in sociotechnical networks of relations (Mort, Roberts, Pols, Domenech, & Moser, 2013). Although engaging with scientific and biomedical information, this relational thinking often at least partially distances itself from expert views. Brown and Michael (2002), for example describe a shift from authority to authenticity in their analysis of publics' assessment of the risks associated with xenotransplantation (the transplantation of living cells, tissues or organs from one species to another). Cox and McKellin (1999) describe a gap between patients' and clinicians' views of who counts as 'family' when considering genetic risk of Huntington's disease. Biomedical knowledge is central to the production of new forms of risk, but does not determine individuals' responses to these (Novas & Rose, 2000).

Our ethnographic studies show that biosensors are framed by manufacturers and consumers as ways to contain and manage risk but also that users almost always find that the biological data provided open up complex health-related questions that experts are unable or unwilling to answer (Kragh-Furbo, Mackenzie, Mort, & Roberts, (2016); Wilkinson, Roberts, & Mort, 2015). Using biosensors in our two research areas – personalised genetic testing and fertility monitoring – then, often leads to participation in online forums in which users collectively attempt to parse the meaning of data and, importantly, to decide what to do to manage their individual risks.

'Lay' people's focus on relationality when considering risk, in our view, indicates a keen awareness of the broader social, political and ethical implications of biomedical risk categories, assessments and related practices. Following users, consumers or patients through their engagement with risk discourses and associated biomedical and other technologies (such as online forums), and asking them to articulate their thoughts and actions in interviews and focus groups, allows researchers to begin to see what these extra-medical considerations might be. But what might we find if we ask a broader population of respondents to tell us what they think about biosensors and their implications for health, risk and society?

Two types of biosensors

Our research addresses two increasingly important areas of biosensing: personalised genetic testing and fertility monitoring. As detailed later, we focus on widely available, relatively affordable biosensors designed and marketed to assist consumers to assess and manage health risks outside of public or private clinical regimes.

Genetic testing

In December 2014 23andMe, a commercial company based in the United States, launched its DTC testing kits in the United Kingdom and subsequently the £125 Saliva Collection Kit and Personal Genome Service went on sale online and over-the-counter at Superdrug stores (BBC, 2014). After spitting into the tube that comes with the kit, customers send their samples to 23andMe's contracted laboratory in California that processes the samples using microarray technologies, and within a few weeks, their testing results are ready to view via email. Heavily criticised by the Royal College of General Practitioners, the Personal Genome Service provides data that claim to show users how their genetic profile may impact their health and how their family history may be implicated in possible future health conditions (The Guardian, 2014a; 2014b). These claims are regarded by many experts as highly dubious. Hardy and Singleton (2009), for example argue in the *New England Journal of Medicine*, results are based on data from genome-wide association studies for common, complex conditions that involve multiple genes with relatively common genetic variants that each confers a modest to small effect on disease risk.

Reacting to the over-the-counter availability of the tests, the Royal College of General Practitioners chair Maureen Baker said their availability could cause unnecessary worry and anxiety, put extra pressure on doctors and that considering a genetic family history:

is a key skill that is best left to medical professionals, who can also provide the necessary support and advice to patients in a private and confidential environment. (Baker cited in The Guardian, 2015)

While 23andMe does not provide counselling as part of its service, the company encourages its customers to contact a healthcare professional, and in effect, as Fiore-Gartland and Neff note, the interpretative work is brought back into the medical system. 23andMe might cut out 'a middleman while integrating seamlessly all the parts of the middleman's very system' (Fiore-Gartland & Neff, 2016). Thus, while the company attempts to disrupt traditional medicine through a so-called democratisation of access to information, the disruption discourses ignore, Fiore-Gartland and Neff argue, the issue of interpretation; data generated by the tests require mediation: forms of interpretative work done by individuals themselves or by medical professionals.

23andMe's UK launch was controversial, sparking much comment in the news media and from the public, since 23andMe had previously been banned from marketing its Personal Genome Service in the United States by the Food and Drugs Administration (FDA) which regulates products intended to diagnose, mitigate, treat or prevent disease, over concerns about the 'public health consequences of inaccurate results from the PGS [Personal Genome Service] service' (FDA, 2013; The Guardian, 2013). In the letter to 23andMe, FDA had expressed concern about the company's failure to demonstrate that its service has been analytically and clinically validated, and noted how 23andMe had suddenly stopped communication with the administration in May 2013 after 4 years of interaction. Later that year, 23andMe launched an aggressive national television, radio and online advertising campaign that is said to have piqued the FDA's interest (WSJ 2013). 23andMe has since worked with the FDA to get its tests analytically and clinically validated for their intended uses, and in October 2015, the company relaunched its Personal Genome Service on the US market with health risk reports that meet the FDA standards.

Fears have also been raised about the misuse of confidential data; 23andMe (which has Google as a major investor) has declared it does not share the individual-level genetic data with insurance companies or any other interested party without a user's explicit consent, unless required by law. However, the company may share a person's anonymised and aggregated data with third parties that include its business partners (23andMe, 2015). While these type of data have been stripped of personal information, it has been demonstrated that 'it is possible, in principle, to identify an individual's genomic data within a large dataset of pooled genomic data' (Vorhaus 2009). This also raises questions about data security. While 23andMe uses 'robust authentication methods to access its database', the company also acknowledges that 'it is never possible to fully guarantee against breaches in security' (23andMe, 2015).

Users of 23andMe are also invited to participate in the company's research. If they consent to 23andMe Research, their individual-level data may be shared with third parties such as pharmaceutical companies and 23andMe may 'create, commercialize, and apply this new knowledge to improve health care' (23andMe, 2015). It did this in 2012, when the company announced its first patent – related to its Parkinson's disease research – that came as a surprise to many of its customers, and while 23andMe 'aim[s] for these discoveries to benefit everyone' (23andMe, 2012), it is unclear who will benefit the most. In their study of 23andMe's research practice, Harris, Wyatt, and Kelly (2012) argued that while 23andMe represents research participation as a form of gift exchange, this framing is used to draw attention away from the free, clinical labour that drives the profitability of 23andMe.

Wyatt, Harris, Adams, and Kelly (2013) analysed the performative dimensions of trust relations between 23andMe and its users, drawing on Shapin and Schaffer's (1985) discussion of material, literary and social technologies. They are sceptical of the ways in which 23andMe tries to build trust with its users, for example by use of personal language (use of 'you'), promotion of links to the National Institute of Health, providing profiles of its advisory board with details of their university affiliations, the use of firewalls, secure online payment systems, encryption of data, lab certifications and others.

Home reproductive technology

Whilst there has been less visible controversy surrounding home reproductive technologies, some of these devices do involve the collection and storage of large amounts of personal biological data with the attendant concerns about accountability and potential commercial use. In this article we consider how having data about ovulation cross cuts into medical protocols around the diagnosis and treatment of infertility.

Companies promise that home ovulation monitoring devices will increase the chances of becoming pregnant and reduce the need for invasive medicine (testing and intervention) (Guardian, 2014c). The Clearblue Fertility Monitor for example, in which urine tests are made to detect changes in hormones, claims to increase the chances of becoming pregnant by 89%. Ovulation microscopes offer saliva-based fertility testing as a way of detecting the surge in oestrogen which occurs before ovulation. If oestrogen is present in saliva, then crystallised ferning patterns will appear on the slide. Other monitors include Ovusense, a vaginal sensor which continuously records a woman's temperature while sleeping, and DuoFertility, also a temperature monitoring sensor worn under the arm. With DuoFertility, users receive a hand-held reader to record additional fertility information such as ovulation pain, sexual intercourse or cervical mucous. A little-known device, the OV-Watch, is a watch-like sensor that records changes in hormone levels found in skin perspiration. In addition to wearable sensors, an increasing number of fertility apps have also become available such as Ovia Fertility or Glow, creating platforms for women to input data about their bodies, again with a view to increasing their chances of becoming pregnant. Of course, sensors and apps work with the body in different ways. Whilst sensors record and detect changes in bodily fluids or temperature, with apps the user must input the data they have produced using their body as a measuring tool. However, both sensors and apps respond to, albeit different forms of, biological matter.

These two different examples of biosensing systems share significant social and ethical dimensions. They both draw on narratives of enhanced visibility and self-optimisation: knowing about your genetic risks brings enhanced responsibility and pressure for behaviour change; knowing your ovulation patterns implies enhanced control of fertility. Both systems draw on 'biologically active agents' sampled at home but which then travel through sociotechnical networks involving laboratory and web spaces, in which they become transformed into data. In this way they come to frame the body as a 'complex information network' (Lupton, 2012) and are both to a varying extent individualising, in the sense that they produce health/fertility as unconnected with wider conditions in society or with public policy. Outside of clinical control and commercially located, they are the subject of severe criticism from medical professionals on grounds of accuracy and effectiveness.

Another recent development which exemplifies the social risks associated with proliferation and commercialisation of 'digital health' is the 'care.data' initiative (NHS England, 2015) which indicates that personal health data (in the United Kingdom arising from the universal health service) is now regarded by government and some industry sectors as a strategic economic resource. Decades of accumulated health and medical data for the population in England and Wales are currently being re-packaged as a globally unique platform for biomedical innovation. The care.data initiative has been particularly controversial since earlier in 2014 as it was revealed that the Government's Health and Social Care Information Centre had sold hospital records covering 47 million citizens, identified by date of birth and postcode, to an insurance organisation (Telegraph, 2014). So even if the NHS continues to be the primary repository for health data in the United Kingdom, it is clear that these data are beginning to circulate more widely. While not associated specifically with biosensors, the security of personal data was a key issue raised by the citizen's panel.

Comment

Biosensing helps users to collect, store and assess personal health-related data. Many biosensors also facilitate the capture and storage of such data by commercial entities. Importantly, all of this labour occurs outside (although sometimes in tandem or conversation with) traditional biomedical networks (e.g. clinician's surgeries, public databases, hospitals), and out with the regulatory processes associated with medical technologies. As increasing numbers of people buy and use these technologies, then, we need to consider the social, ethical and political costs of health monitoring and to think critically about how these technologies re-articulate and re-make health, risk and society.

Methodology

The study we draw on in this article was part of a broader interdisciplinary and multi-institutional, international research programme, 'Biosensors in Everyday Life', supported by Intel's University Research Office (2010–2013). In our part of this programme, we have conducted three interlinked projects under the title 'Living data: making sense of biosensors': a doctoral study on DTC genetic testing; a doctoral study on home fertility monitoring; and the citizens panel 'Our Bodies, Our Data', we draw on in this article.

As we have noted, much of the debate and analysis of biosensing focuses on its technical and scientific base. Given the potential social effects of such technologies we felt that it was important to engage a broader spectrum of voices in developments in the biosciences and management of data where innovations were exposing the public to challenges such as the management of uncertainty and risk, and the extensive circulation of their personal data. We therefore organised a 2-day event, 'Our Bodies, Our Data', in which a carefully selected sample of citizens in Lancashire was invited to interrogate and debate complex issues arising from the introduction of DTC genetic testing and fertility monitoring devices, matters which the public seldom gets chance to consider formally.

We adopted the deliberative panel approach from the citizens' jury model and drew on a now established tradition of participatory democratic practice (Coote & Lenaghan, 1997; Gooberman-Hill, Horwood, & Calnan, 2008; Kashefi & Mort, 2004; Mort, Harrison, & Dowswell, 1999). An overview of methods and case studies in public engagement can be seen at the National Coordinating Centre for Public Engagement site: http://www.publi cengagement.ac.uk/how. If carefully conducted using transparent processes, it can provide opportunities for citizens who are not necessarily involved with, or users of, particular innovations, to learn about them, ask critical questions and respond thoughtfully to the social, ethical and technical questions they provoke. The approach enables the formation of public understandings and opinion to enter a domain dominated by experts. As such, it is a legitimate space within which to identify issues for debate and to offer recommendations to key actors involved in the development, marketing and regulation and consequences of those technologies. As a research method, citizens' panels allow us to move beyond the experience of particular patient groups or interested actors to consider the views of a much broader group of respondents, who are both more implicated than they may have thought they were, but also potentially more able to consider a range of implications without referring to direct personal investment. As suggested earlier, speaking to citizens allows us to focus on the implications of biosensing for society as a whole, raising significant ethical, social and political questions about risk, responsibility, trust and accountability.

We acknowledge that this approach has a number of limitations. While consultation is important, as Boaz, Chambers, and Stuttaford (2014) argue, it does not equate with participation, and runs the risk of allowing 'the research enterprise, health services and governance structures to continue largely with business as usual'. Another important criticism centres on the timing of citizens' engagement. If the engagement takes place 'downstream', then citizens' ability to influence policy or technological development is limited; if too far 'upstream', the process can be frustrating as there are few materialised examples to examine (Pidgeon & Rogers-Hayden, 2007). Additionally in our case, the panel took place in the north-west of England, a location that shaped the outcomes of the consultation in various ways. For example, the participants all clearly identified the National Health Service (NHS) as the primary and most trusted provider of healthcare and health information. It was widely taken for granted that the NHS should also take care of biomedical and health data. This strongly reflects participants' 'history' with publicly funded universal healthcare.

The panel process

The 15-member panel was recruited and organised independently by a consultant experienced in participatory methods, Dr Sue Weldon, to reflect a broad cross-section of citizens, rather than a representative sample of society. Each participant was approached with information about the panel process and if interested, subsequently followed up with a formal informed consent process. Members were recruited, from within a local area of 40 miles, to selection criteria encompassing: gender (broadly equal numbers of men and women); age (from 18 to 75 years); a range of residency including urban and rural, private and social housing; a mix of occupation/education, and diversity in physical ability and ethnicity (see Table 1).

We reimbursed participants' travel expenses and paid them a small fee for their time and all were sent a copy of the draft report for comment. In contrast with ethnographic, interview or focus group-based studies, which concentrate purposively on affected individuals or groups, these were citizens with no professional or vested interest in the technologies to be discussed. They did, however, bring a very wide variety of life experience and knowledge to the consultation. Interestingly, it later emerged that all the panel participants had some connection, either direct or indirect, to the underlying issues brought up in the scenario or debate around biosensing and data, either from personal experience or through family members or friends. This shows how 'innovations' which at first might seem distant from us are in fact embedded in everyday life (Figure 1).

The 'Our Bodies, Our Data' examination of DTC genetic testing and home reproductive technologies was initiated by a scenario entitled the 'Brown Family from

Table 1. The panel.

Name[a]	Age (years)	From	Occupation	Interests
Steve	37	Preston	Charity worker	Football coach
Mary	61	Lancaster	Caterer	Writing and performing
Peter	61	Birmingham	Carer	Health and social care
Stan	45	Morecambe	Unemployed	Volunteering
George	46	Kendal	Disability Service worker	Disability rights; wheelchair user
Carol	18	Morecambe	Casual work	Volunteering
Winston	57	Dominica	Community education worker	Equality issues
Laura	71	Germany	Retired teacher	Languages
Debbie	42	Heysham	Carer	Volunteering with children
Maura	24	Holme	Office worker	First responder
Rhona	28	Bare	Student	Body movement and health
Callum	19	Preston	Volunteer	Astronomy/star gazing
Reg	75	Morecambe	Retired probation officer	Canoeing, sailing, rowing
Dave	67	Preston	Retired aircraft engineer	Trade union movement
Iris	44	Lancaster	Full-time homemaker	Adoption, counselling

[a]These are all pseudonyms and actual identification is protected.

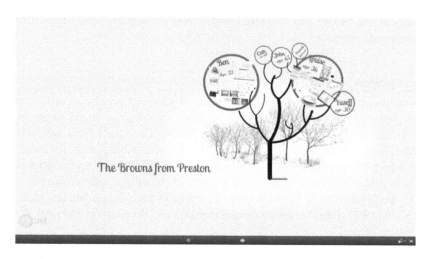

Figure 1. The scenario.

Preston' (Table 2). This fictional family included 32-year-old Ben, who was concerned about his risk of Alzheimer's disease and was engaging with DTC genetic testing, and 36-year-old Louise who was trying to conceive and had purchased fertility monitoring devices. Based on data from the two doctoral ethnographic studies, the scenario explored the reactions of family members to Ben and Louise's engagement with biosensing, and introduced the practicalities of testing and receiving results. The scenarios articulated possible concerns, but were neither positive nor negative about biosensing.

Table 2.   The scenario: the Browns from Preston.

Theresa, Grandmother died at 75 with Alzheimer's disease
John, 65, Theresa's son, becoming forgetful
Cath, 60, John's wife, concerned about her husband and son
Ben, 32, John and Cath's son, single, uses genetic testing kit from 23andMe, found
  to be at 'increased risk of Alzheimer's disease'
Louise, 36, John and Cath's daughter, married, infertility issues, uses ovulation
  microscope
Yusef, 30, Louise's husband, infertility issues
Part 1: Making sense of genetic data

Ben, aged 32, is a single man with a good job working in a small engineering company. He likes computers and his smart phone, and enjoys downloading films and surfing the web. One of his favourite websites recently is called 23andMe. This is a company based in the United States that sells genetic testing kits directly to the public. A friend at work had read about 23andMe in the magazine *Wired* and mentioned it over lunch one day. He had been quite excited about it .... Read more at https://biosensordata.wordpress.com/2015/10/

Scenarios are often used in futures planning or to develop policy where there are a number of possible outcomes. Scenarios are seen as helpful informative tools to work with imagined problems and important concerns. Features of systems can be explored in a variety of ways through the storyline, and can be supplemented by using examples of products, websites and illustrative documents. The idea of using a family scenario in the 'Our Bodies, Our Data' inquiry was to present common features occurring between DTC genetic testing and home reproductive technologies, allowing participants to reflect on the possible day-to-day implications of these, and to act as prompts for discussion and points of departure. The scenario did not deliberately highlight any particular risks: in this article we focus on risk arises from the panel's deliberations.

'Expert' witnesses are frequently used in citizen panel projects to assist members in gaining an understanding of, for example how new technical systems have developed, are supposed to work or what legal or ethical frameworks are relevant to their implementation. By responding to questions developed by groups of panel members, and addressing their concerns about the scenarios, the witnesses share their expertise with panel members. Through this discussion and form of questioning, the gap between lay and expert can be narrowed. The speakers we invited to 'Our Bodies, Our Data' panel discussion provided input from four perspectives: primary healthcare; health research (specifically genetics); patient/user support groups (specifically infertility); NGO/third sector organisations (specifically genetics). The witnesses were a general practitioner and GP tutor/primary care medical educator with additional qualifications in sexual health, obstetrics and gynaecology, contraceptive techniques and paediatrics; the public programmes, manager at a centre for public engagement, education and training in biomedicine with a background in genetic counselling and science education; the chief executive of a national infertility charity dedicated to the support of those affected by infertility; and the director of a pressure campaigning group which specialises in the ethics, risks and social implications of human genetics. In the weeklong period between Day 1 and 2 the panel was invited to reflect on the expert witnesses' responses. Finally, in small self-selected groups the panel developed a series of recommendations: for the biosensor industries; for government, regulators and commissioning agents; and for civil society organisations (NGOs).

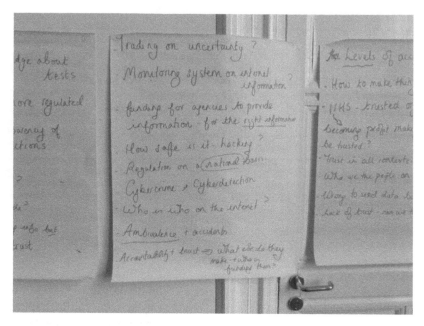

Figure 2.   Panel discussion running notes.

Plenary and group discussions were audio-recorded and transcribed, and all material was anonymised. Analysis began in the final group session of the panel itself and is partly contained within the recommendations for change. Analysis by the authors in terms of theory generation was conducted later from multiple readings of the transcripts and field notes. Later we have used text boxes for 'collective quotes' such as questions generated by small groups of panel members. Other extracts are taken from individual verbatim transcripts, although we have not attributed quotes to particular participants (who are listed in Table 1). We use participants' words to show the views of the panel, not in order to trace any particular view back to a particular participant. In a citizen's panel, members are always speaking within a collective setting, even if expressing personal views. In this article, we show how the citizen panel method produces different forms of data from other qualitative research, forms which include collectively developed questions, discussion summaries written on flip charts/post-it notes, field notes and comments on draft reports, in addition to verbatim transcripts. Here, participants speak as citizens not as representatives of interest groups or as members of particularly affected populations: the aim is to explore questions relevant to all social groups (Figure 2).

The Lancaster University Research Ethics Committee provided approval for the associated doctoral studies of DTC genetic testing and home reproductive technologies on 23 May 2012 and 20 July 2012, respectively.

Findings

Risks identified by the panel

Asking questions about the technologies

Day 1 of the panel meeting began with discussion of issues raised by the scenario; members were interested and concerned to learn that consumers could purchase a service that provided personal genetic information and future health predictions. They also raised questions about the accuracy and usefulness of the data produced in biosensing, and group questions focused on the regulation of biosensing systems. The panel summarised these questions in the following way highlighting potential dangers, such as data security and test errors and the need for measures to enhance trust such as professional scrutiny and state regulation.

Panel's questions for the experts: on trust, reliability and regulation

- What measures are in place to keep the data secure?
- Is there any professional body to scrutinise these products/sites?
- Are these [fertility] products regulated in the United Kingdom?
- What is the quality of genetic tests? Are the results reliable?
- To what extent, for instance, can common conditions such as cancer be tested for?
- Can you tell that you are ovulating from saliva? Aren't there better ways?
- Would you agree that 20,000 readings [of temperature, in relation to ovulation] creates an illusion of accuracy?
- How useful is the information to Ben really?

The panel members were particularly concerned about the relationship between the NHS and the commercial provision of tests/testing kits and several of the questions they articulated referred to the role of the NHS.

Panel's questions for the experts: on relationships with clinicians

- What information (from websites and tests) do people bring to their GP?
- How far should doctors interact with new commercial technologies?

The panel members were very uneasy about commercial motivation of the companies providing the tests and problems this created for protecting the interests of those using the tests as was evident in the following questions:

Panel's questions for the experts: on commercialisation

- Who is going to benefit from the tests?
- Are there links between companies that offer tests and companies that sell drugs?
- Can employers/insurance companies have access to genetic data?

The panel members were concerned about the need for consumer education and whether the companies providing the tests could be trusted as reflected in the following questions:

Panel's questions for the experts: on education and trust

- Is there a need for better education?
- How do we know whether we can trust these companies? Is there a trusted website to make sense of other sites?

They were also very concerned about the effects on the wider family of the longer-term implications of accessing genetic information asking the following questions:

Panel's questions for the experts: on human costs

- How do you cope with the worry/concern for the whole family?
- How can people be supported to cope with the results?

Formulating recommendations

On Day 2, after small group discussion, panel members gathered in a plenary session in which they expressed a high level of concern about the commercial marketing of genetic tests and fertility devices. Some members of the panel questioned whether these were being designed to meet the needs of the consumer or to deliver returns for shareholders. They felt that a business model primarily motivated by profit, rather than one to provide public benefit, could lead to manipulation of markets to create more demand for (sometimes unnecessary or inappropriate) products fuelled by heightened public aware-ness of future risks of genetic conditions or infertility. One participant argued that:

> They (the companies) can set the agenda by creating fear and then, out of this fear, a demand for a service.

Many panel members reflected on current changes in the way health services were being provided in the United Kingdom and noted that the intrusion of commercial interests into their relationship with their general practitioner and in some cases, patient support organisations, had the capacity to undermine their trust in them. 'You trust them more if they are not trying to sell you something', was a typical comment.

Managing and containing uncertainty

Panel members were very concerned with accountability, trust, standards and care of data. In the absence of specific regulation, the panel discussed the need to have some way of assessing the standard of products and services. One repeated suggestion was for a 'kite mark' or symbol to denote a safe product, endorsed by a trusted institution such as the NHS. Another concern was about personal data protection and fears were expressed that, once the data are supplied to a company (online), it would remain indefinitely available to be used in unknown ways.

Trust

The panel members agreed that a person's trust in an organisation, company or product is critical. Trust is built out of knowledge (of the organisation, company or product) and often on the continuity of relationships. Panel members spoke about how trusting relation-ships could be established with doctors, health professionals or even with organisations through experience and over time. One woman expressed concern that digital commu-nications erode that sense of relationship continuity. Many panel members felt that the NHS had always represented a standard of reliable healthcare as a 'trusted organisation', with one participant stating:

> I'd only really trust something that was sponsored by the National Health Service ... because I think the NHS is a trusted organisation which is there to look after us.

Panel members recognised that the NHS was undergoing significant structural change in the direction of privatisation and that this might affect future perceptions of trust. A relevant remark was

> The only problem with that is that in the future, because of all the privatisation, there are going to be a lot of diverse companies involved in making a profit from the NHS and therefore who can we trust in the future?

Accountability

Panel members pointed out that accountability is an essential part of a trusting relationship, and rests on ability to hold individuals or organisations to account through a chain of responsibility. In this context one person referred to the 2013 European 'horse meat scandal' in which supermarkets were selling meat products that were contaminated with horse meat (and other meats). The complexity of the meat supply chain meant that it was difficult to locate the source of contamination. The panel members argued that people could only trust a system if they perceived those operating it were committed to the general good rather than in pursuit of self-interest. One man argued, 'With a doctor you can always go back if he (sic) misdiagnoses you. What happens if the test results are wrong?' whilst another asked:

> What else does 23andME sell? . . . because how do we know they've got the specialists to do the tests? How do we know where the tests are going?

This concern was succinctly expressed by the question: 'How many companies are in the chain?'

The panel members agreed that biosensor technology companies should formulate and publish a set of over-arching values and ethical guidelines. This recommendation arose out of concern that lack of regulation might lead to a fall in standards, particularly in respect of business practice and ethics. Panel members wanted to see written commitments to standards of good practice and argued that these guidelines should include an explicit commitment to develop new biosensor technologies for public benefit. 'This would give you some basis for trusting them, and holding them accountable', one participant stated.

Panel members argued that companies should be transparent and accountable in dealings with the public. They felt that the issue was particularly important when products were marketed online and there might be more than one company or organisation in the chain, obscuring responsibility for the quality, accuracy or safety:

> They need to be accountable about the way they are marketing as well as what they are marketing. So they need to be completely transparent about the product . . . . The people who vouch for it, so called experts . . . . So you want their name, their education, references to their work and so on . . . .

Standards

In the absence of regulation to protect the consumer (when products and services were being marketed in other countries where regulation may be weaker or non-existent), panel members felt that it would be difficult to maintain standards of quality and accuracy in the United Kingdom. They expressed the desire to 'see some qualifications' of those offering a service and suggested:

> This comes back to the [idea about statutory] warning on the packet. You could make it mandatory to give a warning [that results may not be reliable].

Minimal standards of accuracy were not high on the panel's agenda; instead they were concerned that advertising claims made by bionsensor companies were regulated.

Care of data

Panel members expressed concerns about the handling of personal data by companies that might use these data for further research without consent or pass it on to other companies selling treatments and drugs. They discussed the possibility that data might get into the wrong hands and such misuse of data might affect an individual's insurance or employment status. One member expressed this concern very strongly in terms of 'stealing':

> My feeling is that people who want to steal my information are more clever than I am.

Panel members felt that biosensor companies should guarantee to treat personal data respectfully and safely, specifically in offering a choice of consent arrangements. They argued that personal data were precious part of personal identity, where informed consent arrangements were vital. Transparency about what would happen to personal data, and possible future use, would facilitate informed consent arrangements. Summarising group debate, one participant explained:

> So for instance, before buying a service like a [genetic] test, right at the front there would be choices about what's going to happen to your data, whether you consent to any use, some use, or perhaps no use of the data apart from sending the results back to you. At the moment that's not the case, you don't know what they do with the data. There should be guidelines that the company have set up for the use of this data, and they should be published as well as part of telling you what the service is.

Panel members were also concerned about how data could be de-coupled from personal information in order to respect the anonymity of the consumer: 'It seems they all want us to be locked in, and that is a concern for a lot of people'.

Provision of counselling and advice, when considering the wider implications of biosensor test results, was called for. For instance, test results might suggest a need for further treatment, often with implications for other family members. It might be inappropriate for a company to offer counselling but there should be der implications of biosensor test results, was called for. For instance, test results might suggest a need for further treatment, often with implications for other family members. It might be inappropriate for a company to o

Non-governmental support (including charities, patient support groups, disability groups) was needed to help users of biosensors understand and make sense of online purchases, providing independent information and informal counselling. As one member suggested:

> ...so if you did the 23andMe test and found that you had a condition ... to have support networks in place to help you deal with that ... [in the genetic testing scenario] Ben didn't know what to do and 23andMe didn't help ... so someone to talk to about the information and provide support.

The first and most useful role for NGOs would be to provide clear information about what tests, or biosensor services could offer and what they cannot offer. One woman argued that an important role would be in questioning some of the unrealistic claims being made by companies offering tests and biosensor devices:

We want them to provide unbiased facts, or tell us what is missing. I would be looking for facts. What does this do? What does it offer? What are the problems?

It was felt that users might need the guidance of an independent signposting service to direct users to specific support groups: 'They are not going to know where to get this help'.

NGOs could provide a protected space, outside the professional services, for peer support offered by people who had similar experiences to share, in the view of the panel. In the scenario, Ben was confused by the conflicting advice he accessed from an online support group and, although it is normal practice to access such groups, there is little sense of who the forum discussants are, or of their motivations. Such spaces could be 'infiltrated' by companies seeking to promote products. Two essential elements of an authentic forum would be trust and reassurance: 'You want to speak to someone who has been in a similar situation', said one member.

The panel agreed that in the process of undergoing tests or using biosensor monitoring devices, there was a danger of being over-directed or 'channelled' in one direction towards further treatment, for instance with a course of drugs or IVF. They agreed that was a role for patient support groups in providing alternative options so that users would be enabled to make choices. One member said

> [It's about] groups recognising the needs and desires behind decisions people make to have these tests done ... particularly we were talking about their ... need to have or want a child ... so if these groups also acknowledge that need, and recognise that need and perhaps offer alternatives or the support around that need, then perhaps that would give a more balanced experience ...

There was a role for patient or user organisations in offering education about internet safety as an 'antidote' to industry promotion, advertising and unrealistic claims. The panel recognised that advertising could be a powerful way of offering hope, but they noted that it was important to provide a warning and some guidance – particularly for children. A young woman summarised this view in the following way:

> We don't accept anymore our limitations. That you can't always improve on a situation. People will want to have something because they see it advertised ... children ... don't learn how to deal with advertising messages and images.

Discussion in the panel centred on the future relationship between commercial interests and the NHS in respect of 'buying in' services from both public and private providers. Initially, there was much panel debate about how the NHS could take a pro-active role in setting up a self-funded unit to supply data services (in competition with US companies such as 23andMe). Panel members suggested that by building on the ready availability of health data, these services could be used to extend population screening (for such things as breast and bowel cancer) by including genetic information. They suggested that the NHS could then raise much needed revenue by selling services to organisations such as pension groups. However, members also reflected on the dangers of selling information, either to individuals, public bodies (for research) or to organisations. One woman pointed out:

> As a principle, it's your body, your data. It belongs to you. If you want information it should be available (to you) free of charge.

The panel argued that safeguarding personal information and explaining how adequate levels of protection would be maintained could be done through consent arrangements.

They suggested that the choice to 'opt in' rather than 'opt out' of data storage was a safer option. Serious reservations were expressed about the sharing of data records, when such data had been collected from different sources such as screening, health records and numerous other sources such as bone marrow donors. It was felt that such anonymised data could be linked to patient records. One member stated:

> It's all about trusting them to look after your data. Don't lose the opportunity to safeguard this [data].

The panel stressed the need for a greater awareness of 'skilling up' to meet future demands for professional and public information in the area of biosensing. It noted that professional advice and counselling would be vital in understanding what test results mean for individuals and, for the wider public, but there was doubt that most health professionals had the skills to address public concerns about the social and ethical issues and identified the need for training programmes for clinicians in offering information, support and counselling (where necessary). The panel also identified the need for public information (written in lay terms) in primary care centres, schools and public places inviting people to learn more about biosensors such as genetic tests and fertility monitors and what they could offer. The panel wanted a trusted body to act as 'watchdog' in determining which companies are offering reliable information, and to direct people to reliable testing companies. A vetting/monitoring service might determine which websites to trust how to make sense of claims.

Discussion

'Our Bodies, Our Data' was an attempt to move consideration of digital health technologies – specifically the design, development and provision of two kinds of biosensors – from the domain of experts to that of citizens. While some of the views expressed by panel members resonated with those criticisms made by professionals and the third sector (as exemplified above by the Royal College of General Practitioners and the Alzheimer's Society), members also raised wider concerns. These included trust and accountability; effect on family relationships; regulation, standards and scrutiny; expertise and training; data security; exploitation of anxious or vulnerable people; commodification of the body; support and counselling; provision of alternatives and maintenance of publicly funded services.

The introduction and evaluation of biosensors to date has been dominated by individualising manufacturer and user accounts of self-optimisation and responsibilisation. Other researchers (Novas & Rose, 2000; Rabinow, 1999) have shown that genetic discourses do not necessarily individualise (geneticise), but can lead affected individuals to identify as members of biosocial groups such as patient organisations. Whilst existing studies, including our own ethnographic accounts, highlight both the surveillance possibilities and the biosociality implied in much biosensing (e.g. pointing to their entwinement with online discussion forums) (Saukko, 2004; Nafus 2016), 'Our Bodies, Our Data' is engaged with people as citizens rather than as members of an embodied interest group. This engagement necessarily focused on more collective social and policy-related concerns, facilitating the articulation of technology's multiple stories and places and the reimagining of what biosensors might do and mean.

As in existing work on health and risk, questions of relationality were important in our study; people expressed high levels of concern about interpersonal relations. However, they also noted the importance of individuals' actions for others in their communities and indeed for society more broadly. They were concerned, in other words, not only with the ways in which health risks were (or were not) being addressed by biosensing, but with the new social risks associated with personal health monitoring. Members discussed the potential for high levels of anxiety driven by proliferation of information as an increasing risk in contemporary life; debated the importance of trust-building; and displayed skepticism about expert knowledge, recognising the need for interpretation of numbers and demonstrating awareness of recent scandals they saw as relevant such as 'care.data' and horse meat. Not only did the panel members explicitly discuss the relevance of the horse meat scandal for biosensing, their discussion raised issues that were also those highlighted by Regan et al. (2015) in their analysis of the horse meat scandal, who argued that holding individuals and organisations to account would be vital for the rebuilding of trust. The citizen panel approach, in other words, elucidated the social effects of attempts to know and manage future risk through biosensing.

The panel's responses to the dilemmas in the scenarios were informed by the members' multiple embedded perspectives. As such they hold forms of credibility and legitimacy, different from both expert and stakeholders' views. Their recommendations emanate also from a wariness of exploitation and also a concern for social solidarity which is missing from the discourse of the biosensor industry, where benefits are framed in the case of DTC genetic testing at an individual risk level, or in the case of home ovulation monitoring at the level of the couple-as-unit. The panel reflected concern for what kind of society is being made when genetic testing and home reproductive biosensors are promoted and sold to members of the public online or in pharmacies outside of any clinical relationship or service.

Conclusion

Although sometimes invited to participate in research as members of specific affected groups, individuals rarely gain opportunities to debate and express concerns about sociotechnical change *as citizens*. Speaking as a group formed only for the purpose of this research, the panel clearly identified a range of individual, familial and social risks involved in health biosensing developing specific recommendations for governments, technology companies and NGOs. Significantly, they strongly pressed for governmental regulation of biosensing technologies and for informed (NGO and governmental) oversight and care around the promises made and the data produced through these devices. In the ideal society articulated by this panel, biosensing would not remain in a commercial realm populated by keen users and profit-oriented developers, but would be part of a more thoughtful and cautious intersection between state health systems, health activism and responsible innovation. Whilst this finding could be described as idealistic, we argue that it articulates a politically, socially and ethically important desire for a different materialization of health, risk and society.

Acknowledgements

The study underpinning this paper is part of a broader interdisciplinary and multi-institutional, international research programme, Biosensors in Everyday Life, supported by Intel's University Research Office (2010–2013). In our part of this programme, we have conducted three interlinked projects under the title 'Living data: making sense of biosensors': a doctoral study on DTC genetic testing; a doctoral study on home fertility monitoring; and the citizens panel 'Our Bodies, Our Data', reported here.

Disclosure statement

No potential conflict of interest was reported by the authors.

References

23andMe. (2012), *Announcing 23andMe's First Patent*, Retrieved from http://blog.23andme.com/news/announcements/announcing-23andmes-first-patent/ [accessed September 5, 2014]

23andMe. (2015), *Privacy and data protection*, Retrieved from https://www.23andme.com/privacy/ [accessed November 22, 2015]

BBC. (2014), *Controversial test comes to UK*, Retrieved from http://www.bbc.co.uk/news/science-environment-30285581, 2 December, accessed 4 December, 2015.

Boaz, A., Chambers, M., & Stuttaford, M. (2014). Public participation: More than a method? *International Journal of Health Policy and Management*, *3*(5), 291–293. doi:10.15171/ijhpm.2014.102

Brown, N., & Michael, M. (2002). From authority to authenticity: The changing governance of biotechnology, Health. *Risk & Society*, *4*(3), 259–272. doi:10.1080/1369857021000016623

Coote, A., & Lenaghan, E. (1997). *Citizens juries: Theory into practice*. London: Institute for Public Policy Research.

Cox, S., & McKellin, W. (1999). There's this thing in our family': Predictive testing and the construction of risk for huntington's disease'. In P. Conrad & J. Gabe (Eds.), *Sociological perspectives on the New Genetics* (pp. 121–145). London: Blackwell.

FDA. (2013). *Inspections, compliance, enforcement, and criminal investigations*. Retrieved March 31, 2015 from http://www.fda.gov/ICECI/EnforcementActions/WarningLetters/2013/ucm376296.htm

Fiore-Gartland, B., & Neff, G. (2016). Disruption and the political economy of biosensor data. In D. Nafus (Ed.), *Quantified: Biosensing technologies in everyday life* (pp. 101–123). Cambridge: MIT Press.

Gooberman-Hill, R., Horwood, J., & Calnan, M. (2008). Citizens' juries in planning research priorities: Process, engagement and outcome. *Health Expectations*, *11*, 272–281. doi:10.1111/hex.2008.11.issue-3

Hallowell, N. (2006). Varieties of suffering: Living with the risk of ovarian cancer. *Health Risk & Society*, *8*(1), 9–26. doi:10.1080/13698570500532322

Hardy, J., & Singleton, A. (2009). Genomewide association studies and human disease. *New England Journal of Medicine*, *360*(17), 1759–1768. doi:10.1056/NEJMra0808700

Harris, A., Wyatt, S., & Kelly, S. E. (2012). The Gift of Spit (and the obligation to return it). *Information Communication and Society*, *16*(2), 236–257. doi:10.1080/1369118X.2012.701656

Kashefi, E., & Mort, M. (2004). Grounded citizens' juries: A tool for health activism? *A Tool for Health Activism?' Health Expectations*, *7*, 290–302. doi:10.1111/hex.2004.7.issue-4

Kragh-Furbo, M., Mackenzie, A., Mort, M., & Roberts, C. (2016). 'Do biosensors biomedicalize? Sites of negotiation of DNA-based biosensing data practices'. In D. Nafus (Ed.), *Quantified: biosensing technologies in everyday life*. Camb Mass: MIT Press.

Lupton, D. (2012). M-health and health promotion: The digital cyborg and surveillance society. *Social Theory & Health*, *10*(3), 229–244. doi:10.1057/sth.2012.6

Lupton, D. (2015). Towards critical digital health studies: Reflections on two decades of research in health and the way forward. *Health*, *20*(1). doi: 10.1177/1363459315611940

Mort, M., Harrison, S., & Dowswell, T. (1999). Public health panels in the UK: Influence at the margins? In U. A. Khan (Ed.), *Participation beyond the ballot box. European case studies in state-citizen political dialogue* (pp. 94–109). London: Routledge.

Mort, M., Roberts, C., Pols, J., Domenech, M., & Moser, I. (2013). Ethical implications of home telecare for older people: A framework derived from a multi-sited participative study. *Health Expectations*, *18*(3), 438–449. doi:10.1111/hex.12109

Nafus, D. (2013). The data economy of biosensors. In M. J. McGrath & C. N. Scanaill (eds.), *Sensor technologies: Healthcare, wellness, and environmental application*. New York, NY: ApressOpen.

Nafus, D. (2016). Introduction. In D. Nafus (Ed.), *Quantified: biosensing technologies in everyday life*. Camb Mass: MIT Press.

NHS England. (2015). *The care.data programme - Collecting information for the health of the nation*. Retrieved from http://www.england.nhs.uk/ourwork/tsd/care-data/

Novas, C., & Rose, N. (2000). Genetic risk and the birth of the somatic individual. *Economy and Society, 29*(4), 485–513. doi:10.1080/03085140050174750

OED. (2011). *Third Edition (March 2007) - new entry; OED Online version* September 2011

Pidgeon, N., & Rogers-Hayden, T. (2007). Opening up nanotechnology dialogue with the publics: Risk communication or 'upstream engagement'? *Health Risk & Society, 9*(2), 191–210. doi:10.1080/13698570701306906

Rabinow, P. (1999). Artificiality and enlightenment: From sociobiology to biosociality. In M. Biagioli (Ed.), *The science studies reader*. New York, NY: Routledge.

Regan, A., Marcy, A., Shan, L. C., Walls, P., Barnett, J., & McConnon, A. (2015). Conceptualising responsibility in the aftermath of the horsemeat adulteration incident: An online study with Irish and UP consumers. *Health Risk & Society, 17*(2), 149–167. doi:10.1080/13698575.2015.1030367

Roberts, C., & Franklin, S. (2004). Experiencing new forms of genetic choice: Findings from an ethnographic study of preimplantation genetic diagnosis. *Human Fertility, 7*(4), 285–293. doi: 10.1080/14647270400016449

Saukko, P. (2004). 'Genomic susceptibility-testing and pregnancy: Something old, something new'. *New Genetics and Society, 23*(3), 313–325. doi:10.1080/1463677042000305075

Shapin, S., & Schaffer, S. (1985). *Leviathan and the air-pump: Hobbes, boyle, and the experimental life*. Princeton: Princeton University Press.

Telegraph. (2014). Retrieved from http://www.telegraph.co.uk/news/health/news/10656893/Hospital-records-of-all-NHS-patients-sold-to-insurers.html (accessed 31 March 2015)

The Guardian. (2013). *FDA orders genetics company 23andMe to cease marketing of screening service*. Retrieved from http://www.theguardian.com/science/2013/nov/25/genetics-23andme-fda-marketing-pgs-screening (accessed 31 March 2015)

The Guardian. (2014a). *23andMe admits FDA order 'significantly slowed up' new customers*. Retrieved from http://www.theguardian.com/technology/2014/mar/09/google-23andme-anne-wojcicki-genetics-healthcare-dna, 9 March

The Guardian. (2014b) *DNS screening test launches in UK after US ban*. Retrieved from http://www.theguardian.com/technology/2014/dec/02/google-genetic-testing-23andme-uk-launch (2 December accessed 31 March 2015)

The Guardian. (2014c). *Want to get pregnant? There's an App for that*, Retrieved from http://www.theguardian.com/technology/2014/may/18/desperate-pregnancy-app-smartphone-technology-couples-infertility

The Guardian. (2015) *Superdrug criticised by doctors for stocking genetic self-testing kits*. Retrieved from http://www.theguardian.com/science/2015/mar/31/superdrug-criticised-doctors-genetic-self-testing-kits, 31 March (accessed 27 April 2015)

The Wall Street Journal. (2013). *23andMe stops Genetic Test Marketing*. Retrieved from http://www.wsj.com/articles/SB10001424052702304579404579234503409624522 December 2, 2013 [accessed November 23, 2015]

Viseu, A., & Suchman, L. (2010). Wearable augmentations: Imaginaries of the informed body. In J. Edwards, P. Harvey, & P. Wade (Eds.), *Technologised images, technologised bodies* (pp. 161–184). Oxford: Berghahn Books.

Vorhaus, D. (2009). *Re-identification and its Discontents.*, Retrieved from http://www.genomicslawreport.com/index.php/2009/10/13/re-identification-and-its-discontents/ [accessed November 22, 2015]

Wilkinson, J., Roberts, C., & Mort, M. (2015). Ovulation monitoring and reproductive heterosex: Living the conceptive imperative? *Culture Health & Sexuality, 17*(4), 454–469. doi:10.1080/13691058.2015.1005671

Wyatt, S., Harris, A., Adams, S., & Kelly, S. E. (2013). Illness online: Self-reported data and questions of trust in medical and social research. *Theory, Culture & Society, 30*, 131–150. doi:10.1177/0263276413485900

Index